EMERGENCY SURGERY
– Handbook

I0490359

Dr. Sunder Goyal

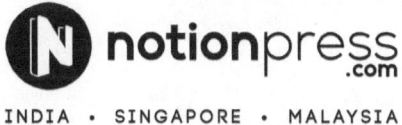

INDIA · SINGAPORE · MALAYSIA

Notion Press

No.8, 3rd Cross Street,
CIT Colony, Mylapore,
Chennai, Tamil Nadu – 600004

First Published by Notion Press 2020
Copyright © Dr. Sunder Goyal 2020
All Rights Reserved.

ISBN 978-1-64850-977-3

Dedicated to

My PARENTS-Sh. Lakhmi Chand Ji & Smt. Kesar Devi JI

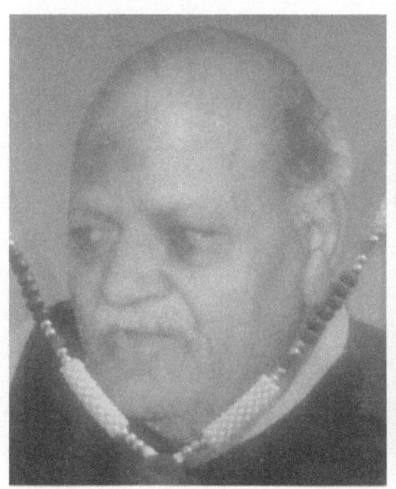 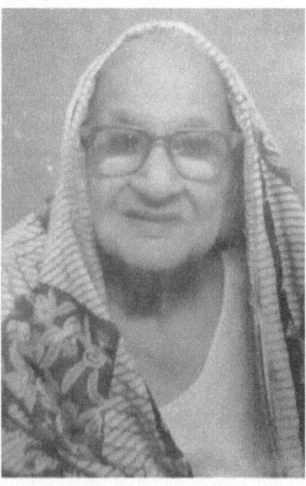

CONTENTS

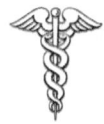

PREFACE

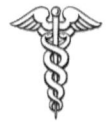

The first edition of this **"Handbook - Emergency Surgery"** provides a brief and useful account of the essential features of the emergency surgical disorders. Adding one more pocket book of emergency surgery to the already existing plethora of books on surgery-needs justification. This small hand book is not intended to be a substitute for standard text book on emergency surgery but is intended an additional help in -emergency- as author has included a) wound care b) sutures and needle c) drains/catheter d) antibiotics e) Fluids & Electrolytes-essential requirements of an emergency surgery. Only in this small book, operating surgeon can refer all these essentials topics for proper management of surgical emergency. Second most important chapter in this book is "How to minimise postoperative wound dehiscence (Pearls of Wound Closure) to decrease the embracing situation for operating surgeon.

The book covers basic principles, as well as provides essential information on diagnosis and management of acute surgical conditions along with preoperative and postoperative patient care. The text covers the field of general surgery but also covers the basic needs of the undergraduate as far as the surgical specialities are concerned. This handbook covers newer topic like abdominal compartment syndrome, Emergency Diagnostic laparoscopy in acute abdomen and Nanotechnology in medicine. This is a unique book which describe the role of pathologist and anaesthetist in acute surgical emergencies.

Value of a book is gauged by utility and uniqueness. Utility of this handy book is due to availability of important chapters like fluids & electrolytes, nutrition, suture & needles and antibiotics in a concise manner at a glance because these topics are very important in preoperatively as well as postoperatively period. All these chapters can be referred immediately and thus saves time of surgeon and helps in management of patients during Golden Hour.

Uniqueness of this handbook is due to simple language of all chapters. This book includes work like Abdominal compartment syndrome (ACS) as abdominal hypertension is important for infusion of all internal organs and multiorgan failure. This book has dealt preoperative and postoperative care in details to decrease morbidity in patients. Despite many advances in surgical techniques, equipment and supplies, complications after abdominal wall closure remain a persistent problem. The ideal abdominal closure should be efficient, provide strength, and serve as a barrier to infection. It should have low rates of fascial dehiscence, infection, hernia formation, suture sinus formation, and pain. Decreasing local wound complications and incisional hernia formation after abdominal wound closure remains a persistent challenge. This book has defined Pearls of wound closure to minimize postoperative wound dehiscence which is a deadly complication and effect physical and mental health of patients as well as of operative surgeon as said by-*"There are few things more embarrassing to a surgeon than the sight of his recently operated patient, his abdomen gaping, and the gut spilling out all around…" ....Moshe Schein*

"Cutting Requires Sharp Instruments,

Shutting of Wound Requires Experience"

Dr Sunder Goyal

"We dedicate this book to our students

who inspire us with their passion for learning

and to our practicing surgical colleagues who share their knowledge

to provide the finest surgical acumen for ailing humans beings"

ACKNOWLEDGEMENTS

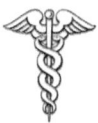

The Future belongs to those

Who believe-in the beauty of their dreams.

Eleanor Roosevelt

To all contributing Authors for their support and cooperation.

To my beloved family members who spared time to help me for completion of this book. Without their cooperation it was impossible to complete this book.

To Dr Sushil Gupta's help for many valuable additions in the book like "Take Home Messages"

To my sweet brother like friend Mr. C.L. Mago ji who was always ready to help.

I am really in debt to my Dean Dr Asim Das for providing me sufficient support to complete this book.

FORWARD

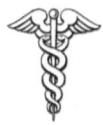

The Hand book of Emergency Surgery is a true 'Vade mecum' or 'Enchiridion' for the intended user (interns, junior Residents, Senior Residents, Casualty Medical Officers) the consultants in the making.

This hand book is not an alternative to the Text Book of Surgery but like the latin words *Vade mecum* or Enchiridion whose literal meaning is "go with me: and as not easily understood by the general public unless explained ... so is the vast knowledge available to the budding surgeons, who is at a loss when he fathoms in the unknown sphere trying to reach the correct destination while working on the patient.

The Unique features in this book are

    a. The humane aspect of surgery framed as guidelines for an ethical practice.

    b. New topics like the abdomen compartment syndrome explained in a easy way.

c. Highlighting the role of the pathologists and Anesthetist in acute abdominal emergencies.

d. Concise and simple manner of presentation of information of fluids and electrolytes, nutrition, use of sutures and needles and antibiotics.

Dr. Sundar Goyal's handbook of surgery will find acknowledgement for his painstaking effort like his contribution has helped in establishment of the Dept. of Surgery at ESIC Medical College Faridabad.

Wish all the readers enrichment of their knowledge.

Prof (Dr) Asim Das

Dean

ESIC Medical College and Hospital

Faridabad, Haryana

FORWARD

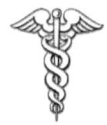

It gives me immense pleasure to write this foreword to **"Emergency Surgery – Handbook".** In today's world majority of medical students use internet to access necessary information. With a click, they get connected to any book. In addition, online textbooks, videos, lectures, demonstrations, simulator applications which are easily available. In spite of all this, good books are always in demand.

I have gone through some of the chapters and found that they are of great use in day to day practice. In addition, this book has adequately illustrated important issues with high quality diagram. Because of its simplicity and adequate coverage of the subjects, this book will be an asset for the students. The chapters cover most of the essential and common aspects of surgery.

This book provides latest and up to date information on different surgical aspects which are important for the students in a surgical ward. Prof. Sunder Goyal has made appreciable attempt to provide the students a comprehensive guide for clear understanding of the subject. I congratulate him on his brilliant efforts and wish him all the success in his endeavours.

Having known Prof. Sunder Goyal for the past 40 years, I have great admiration for his wealth of knowledge in the subject of surgery. This book will be of an enormous help to both undergraduate as well as postgraduate students in surgery. I wish the book a great success.

Dr Sham Lal Singla

Pro-Vicechancellor Provice-Chancellor

SGT University, Gurugram

FORWARD

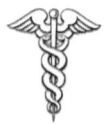

There was paucity of a ready reckoner for residents of surgery which has largely been accomplished by this book brought out with great efforts of Dr. sunder Lal Goyal. He is a well-known surgeon who has established his roots during surgical training only. This book is a reflection of his devotion to academics and a keen desire to train residents of surgery so that they become accomplished surgeons. In the modern times of super specializations, majority is forgetting the basics which are undoubtedly so essential to move forward on the ladder of success. It may not be wrong to state that the book has served its purpose of bringing "back to basics".

Surgical training is a holistic training and not only on mastery of operations. Majority of the present day residents are possibly getting a hazy picture of this hard fact. This book gives a good idea of pre-operative medication, pre and post-operative fluid management, Anesthesia, instrumentation, antibiotics etc. It is a "to the point" book and take home messages are narrated at the need of each chapter. I sincerely hope that this book will be of immense utility to the surgical residents as a ready reckoner.

Dr. Pradeed Garg

MS, MNAMS, DNB, FICS

Senior Professor of Surgery

PGIMS, Rohtak

LIST OF CONTRIBUTORS

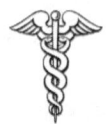

Dr Sham Singla MS (Surgery) Chapter -2
Pro Vice-Chancellor
SGT University, Gurugram, Haryana

Dr Jagdish Dureja MD (Anaesthesia), FNB Critical Care Medicine
Director
KCGMC, Karnal, Haryana

Dr Yamni MS (Surgery)
Director
SHKM Govt Med College, Nuh, Mewat

Dr Nivesh Agarwal MS (Surgery)
Professor Head Surgery Department
KCGMC, Karnal, Haryana

Dr Parveen k. Malik MD (Medicine) FIMSA, PG Diploma Echo

Associate Professor

ESIC Medical College & Hospital, NIT, Faridabad

Member of API, RSSDI, ISCCM, IAE

Dr Pardeep Garg MS (Surgery)

Professor Surgery

Pt BD Sharma PGI Rohtak, Haryana

Dr M.K Garg MS (Surgery)

Prof & Head Surgery

BPS Women Govt. Medical College, Khanpur, Sonepat, Haryana.

Dr Parveen Bhatia MS, FRCS (Eng) FICS, FIAGES (Hon), FMSA,FAIS (Hon) FCLS

Medical DirectorBhatia Global Hospital and Endosurgery Institute

Senior Consultant surgeon

Institute of Minimal Access, Metabolic & Bariatric Surgery , Institute of Robotic Surgery

Sir Ganga Ram Hospital

New Delhi

Dr Gopal Singal MS

Director

Mahararaja Agrasen Medical College

Agroha, Haryana

Dr Ranabir Pal MD (Community Medicine), PhD, MBA, DCH,CMCL-FAIMER Fellow

Professor PSM

MKG Medical College & LSK Hospital

Kishanganj, Bihar

Dr Vandana MD (Gynae &Obst), DNB

Fellowship minimally invasive surgery

Certified Robotic Console Surgeon

Rajiv Gandhi Cancer Institute

Rohini, New Delhi

Dr Snigdha Goyal MD (Pathology)

Consultant Pathologist, HCMS

Panchkula, Haryana

Dr Gaurav Thami MS (Surgery)

Associate Professor Surgery

KCGMC, Karnal, Haryana

Dr Ravi Garg MS, M.Ch.(Paed Surgery)

Assistant Professor

Pediatric Surgery

Govt. Medical College & Hospital, Patiala

Dr Nishant Gurnani MS, M.Ch. Urology)

Assistant Professor

ESIC Med College & Hospital, NIT, Faridabad

Dr Anil Kumar MS (Surgery)

Assistant Professor

ESIC, Med College & Hospital, NIT, Faridabad

Dr Sunder Goyal MS, MNAMS, FAIS, FICS, Diplomate Uro (London)

Prof & Head Surgery

ESIC Med College & Hospital, NIT, Faridabad

Dr Sonia PhD

Department of Food & Technology

Faridabad

Chapter 1

WOUND CARE

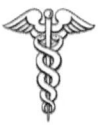

Sunder Goyal

Every surgeon has to deal with wound healing - traumatic or operative. Usually wounds heal through primary intention, if they are not infected. So it is the duty of a surgeon to create the conditions which help in either avoiding the infection or controlling the infection.

The following conditions are required to control the infection, i.e.:

a. Dressing/Drains/Sutures/Needles/Staples/ Antibiotics

b. Good nutrition

c. Fluids and electrolyte balance

d. Correction of anaemia - by blood and blood products

e. Oxygenation

f. No hypotension (shock)

WOUNDS AND DRESSINGS

There are three distinct stages of tissue injury and healing (repair)

1. Stage 1 (Inflammation) -1 to 5 days

2. Stage 2 (Proliferation of collagen and scar formation) - 5 to 14 days

3. Stage 3 (Scar maturation/contraction/ remodelling) This phase is variable and depends upon the nature of the tissue - 4 to 6 weeks. Wound regains 50% of tensile strength at 4 weeks and 70 to 95% in 6 to 8 weeks.

4. Stage 4 (Epithelialization of sutured wound) starts after 48 hours (2 days)

Various types of wounds:

- Clean wounds

- Clean contaminated wounds

- Contaminated wounds

- Infected wounds

Factors affecting wound healing:

- Age

- Weight

- Anemia

- Smoking

- Malnutrition

- Dehydration

- Blood supply

- Foreign body

- Infection/sepsis

- Immune responses

- Chronic illness/Diabetes

- Drugs and radiation therapy

VARIOUS TYPES OF WOUND HEALING

Primary Intension – means surgical wound closure with sutures within 4–6 hours after incision/injury. Healing occurs with minimal oedema, minimal discharge and no bacterial infection.

Secondary Intension – wound edges are left open to heal by granulation, contraction and epithelialization over a period of weeks by changing the dressings frequently. This method is used for clean contaminated wounds.

Tertiary Intension – It is also termed as delayed primary closure. Wound edges are left open after debridement and the dressing is changed frequently till granulation tissue forms. After 4–6 days the edges are surgically re-approximated under sterile conditions after the formation of granulation tissue. Here, unlike secondary intention, the wound is closed with delayed suturing, rather than allowed to close entirely by granulation and epithelialization.

TYPES OF WOUND DRESSINGS

We cannot assess the therapeutic value or ability of available wound dressings, so their contribution to wound healing cannot be ratified. Wound discharge neutralises the antibiotics infused in dressings and thus antibiotics do not penetrate the deeper layers of wounds and are no direct help in wound healing.

The perfect wound dressing should have the following features:

- Mechanical barrier

- Antibacterial function

- Keep the wound hydrated

- Permit fluid exchange and air flow

- Non-sticky by nature

- Painless, nontoxic, hypoallergenic and sterile in nature

- Absorb wound discharge and offensive smell

- Cost effective and available in all sizes

    1. Standard dressings consist of gauze and bandages, non-adhesive meshes, membranes and foils, foams, and tissue adhesives.

    2. Moisture-retaining dressings consist of pastes, creams and ointments, non-permeable or semipermeable membranes or foils, hydrocolloids, hydrogels, and combination products.

    3. Bioactive dressings consist of antimicrobial dressings, single-component biologic dressings.

    4. Skin substitutes consists of epidermal substitutes, autologous and allogenic skin, and skin substitutes containing living cells

TYPES OF DRESSINGS

Amorphous Hydrogels

These cause autolytic debridement of the dead tissue. Ideally they should not be applied to the skin around the wound as gel can result in skin maceration. These dressings are available in tubes, foil packets and spray bottles.

Hydrogel Dressings

Hydrogels are used for pressure ulcers, skin tears, surgical wounds and burns. This dressing can absorb only 5% of wound exudate and is used for dry wounds. It can be used to fill dead space in a large wound.

Hydrocolloid Dressings

These dressings do not permit water, oxygen, or bacteria into the wound as these are occlusive in nature and thus help in the creation of new angiogenesis and healthy granulation tissue. These dressings change pH to acidic and thus stop bacterial growth. These dressings result in autolytic wound debridement and thus help in wound healing.

Alginate Dressings

An alginate is used in infected and non-infected wounds with moderate to heavy exudate as it is capable of absorbing up to 20 times its weight in fluid. It should not be used with dry wounds or wounds with minimal drainage as it could dehydrate the wound and thus delay wound healing.

Composite Dressings

Composite dressings have multiple layers and are useful for wounds with very high exudate. Composite dressings should be avoided if the patient is dehydrated or has delicate skin (children, for instance).

Transparent Films

Transparent film dressings are flexible, transparent, semipermeable polyurethane sheets coated with an acrylic adhesive. They adapt easily to the patient's body surface and contour. The wound can be easily observed due to transparency and they cause autolytic debridement of necrotic wounds.

Table showing types of dressings:

Wound Type	Aim	Dressings
Infected wound with high discharge	Remove necrotic material and absorb discharge	Hydrocolloid, Hydrogels. Alginates for lysis slough and for healthy granulation
Infected wound with low exudate	Autolysis of slough and absorb discharge	Hydrogels. Hydrocolloids
Bad smelling wound	Reduce odour, absorb exudate	Foam or alginate with activated charcoal

If the dressing is done in the operation theatre, then dry dressing is applied. Remove gauze dressing after 48 hours if not soiled.

The solution is used to moisten the deep layer of sterile gauze and includes normal saline and dilute Savlon solution.

COMMONLY USED SOLUTIONS AND OINTMENTS

- Normal saline—used for wounds with healthy granulation tissue

- Diluted Savlon—for clean contaminated wound

- Povidine-Iodine—Antimicrobial, used for grossly contaminated wounds. But, if they are used for a long period they interfere with wound healing

- Silver Nitrate (0.5%)—Antimicrobial, used for 2nd degree and 3rd degree burn wounds. They cause Hyponatremia and Hypochloraemia

OTHER AGENTS USED IN WOUND HEALING

- Collagenase—useful as enzymatic debridement in the treatment of chronic or acute wounds. Usually an antimicrobial ointment is also used in combination.

- Epidermal Growth Factor (EGF)—promotes proliferation and chemotaxis of inflammatory cells.

- Platelet-Derived Growth Factor (PDGF)—promotes proliferation, chemotaxis and collagenase production.

- Transforming Growth Factor Beta (TGF-Beta)—promotes the proliferation of inflammatory cells and fibrosis.

Antibacterial Dressings (Used in locally infected wounds)

1. Aquacel Ag
2. Arglaes
3. Advance
4. Inadine
5. Iodoflex
6. Iodosorb
7. Metrotop Gel

In the management of burns, silver (in the form of silver sulfadiazine cream) is a useful antimicrobial agent.

Currently, Iodine dressings are being used for acute and chronic wound management. Clinically they are mainly used in one of two formats: *(a)* Povidone *(b)* Cadexomer iodine

Cadexomer iodine has good absorptive power: 1 g of Cadexomer iodine can absorb up to 7 ml of fluid. There is a gradual release of iodine in the wound as the exudate is absorbed and thus debrides the wound and reduces the bacterial load. Thyroid function should be monitored in patients who are treated with iodine dressings over a prolonged period.

Metronidazole gel is often used for the control of odour caused by anaerobic bacteria. This is particularly useful in the management of fungating malignant wounds like Diabetic Foot. It may be used alone or as an adjunct to other dressings.

DRAWBACKS OF DRESSINGS

1. Maceration of the skin surrounding a wound.

2. Disruption of healthy tissue on the wound surface due to the use of a highly absorptive dressing on a dry wound.

3. Allergic reactions: Adhesive tapes which keep dressings in place may cause skin allergy.

Take Home Message

The selection of dressing should be such that it absorbs wound discharge and helps in complete healing.

REFERENCES

1. Vanessa Jones, [1] Joseph E Gray, and Keith G Harding. Wound dressings. BMJ. Apr 1, 2006; 332 (7544): 777–780.

2. Choucair M, Phillips T. A review of wound healing and dressing material. Skin and Aging 1998;6:(suppl): 37-43.

3. Hermans MH, Bolton LL. Air exposure versus occlusion: merits and disadvantages of different dressings. J Wound Care 1993;2: 362-5.

4. Morgan DA. Wound management products in the drug tariff. Pharmaceutical Journal 1999;263: 820-5.

5. Thomas S, Leigh IM. Wound dressings. In: Leaper DJ, Harding KG, eds. Wounds: biology and management. Oxford: Oxford University Press, 1998:166-83.

6. Turner TD. Development of wound management products in chronic wound care. In: Krasner D, Rodeheaver G, Sibbald RG, eds. Chronic wound care: a clinical source book for healthcare professionals. 3rd ed. Wayne, PA: HMP Communications, 2001.

7. Winter G. Formation of scab and the rate of epithelialisation of superficial wounds in the skin of the young domestic pig. Nature 1962;193: 293-4. [PubMed]

8. Vermeulen H, Ubbink D, Goossens A, de Vos R, Legemate D. Dressings and topical agents for surgical wounds healing by secondary intention. Cochrane Database Syst Rev 2005;(4): CD003554. [PubMed]

Chapter 2

DRAINS, TUBES AND CATHETER

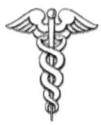

**Dr. Sham Lal Singla[1]; Dr. Sowbir Some[2];
Dr. (Col) M.S. Ray [3]**

INTRODUCTION

Hippocrates described the use of tubes and linens to drain infection from the empyema. Theodore Billroth also believed that drainage of the peritoneal cavity was essential for saving the lives of patients after gastrointestinal surgery. As early as 1940s & 1950s, closed system drains (sealed from atmosphere) and open drains (open to the atmosphere) were introduced. Rubber, Plastic, Polyvinyl chloride (PVC) and silicone were popular materials for drainage in the 20th century & still continue to be in use today.

A Drain is supposed to drain an unwanted collection. It is an appliance or piece of material that acts as a channel for the escape of fluid. It removes secretions, blood and lymph that accumulates in the surgical dead space. Drainage reduces pressure on adjacent organs & vessels enhancing wound perfusion, improve healing and decrease pain. In addition, they may serve as indicator of an anastomotic leak in a contaminated surgery.

In 1940s-60s, the dictum in surgery used to be – "When in doubt use drain." This changed in 1980s "When in doubt, don't use drain." Now it has achieved a controversial status. Where to drain or not to drain is purely governed by the individual judgement and preference of the operating surgeon. To drain or not to drain an area should be totally dictated by the pathology involved in a surgical situation. Often it is better to swallow ones pride and use a drain than not to use one and repent! Basically – a drain drains the muck and does not drain the ego of the surgeon.

However, a Drain is a double edged weapon. It can act like a foreign body. It serves as a conduit for bacteria into the wound and increases the risk of surgical site infection (SSI). It may cause bowel fistulation and disruption of bowel anastomosis.

Effectivity of a Drain: The flow through a hollow structure is expected to follow Hagen-Poiseulle equation:

$$\text{Flow Rate} = \frac{\pi \times (\text{pressure difference}) \times (\text{tube radius})^4}{8 \times \text{fluid viscosity} \times \text{tube length}.}$$

Effectivity of a drain is based on the following factors:

Factors	Flow Rate
Pressure difference	Greater the difference, more the flow
Tube Radius	Bigger the diameter, more is the flow
Tube Length	Shorter the tube, more is the flow
Viscosity	More viscous fluids demand a larger diameter tube

IDEAL DRAIN

There is no ideal drain till date which fits in for all situations.

i. It should be firm, not too rigid, so as to minimize pressure on the adjacent structures.

ii. It should not be too soft either, as it may twist or kink or become blocked.

iii. It should be thermolabile, i.e. it softens inside the body with body temperature to minimize pain and foreign body sensation.

iv. It should be smooth so as not to allow fibrin to adhere on to it and also to allow easy removal.

v. Material should be resistant to decomposition or disintegration so as to avoid leaving behind any part as a foreign body.

vi. Preferably a drain should be siliconized internally to prevent easy blockage by effluents.

vii. It should be non electrolytic, non carcinogenic and non-thrombogenic when used in vascular surgery.

viii. An ideal drain does not exist in practice but effort should be made to choose the most appropriate drain depending upon the situation.

[1]Professor of Surgery & Pro-Chancellor, [2]PG Student, [3]Professor of Surgery,

SGT Medical College, Hospital & Research Institute, Budhera, Gurugram, Haryana.

PURPOSE OF A DRAIN

i. Obliteration of dead space by drainage of unwanted, accumulated fluids like pus, blood, serum lymph, bile or gas.

ii. Continuous drainage to prevent the potential collection of fluids or gases.

iii. Provide a channel for irrigation of serous lined cavities, joint spaces etc., thus removing the nidus for infection.

iv. To create a controlled fistula. e.g.

- After common bile duct exploration use of T-Tube to create "Tubo-choledocho-cutaneous fistula".

- Use of Foley's catheter for "Tubo-Duodenostomy" (Tubo-dudeno-cutaneous fistula) as a "safety valve" to avoid "Duodenal Blow-out" of a diseased duodenum.

    v. To know the precise amount & colour of drainage.

    vi. Crucial watch for excessive bleeding or bile leak to provide early warning of complication.

    vii. To enhance drainage of exudates from the wound

    viii. To help collapse the raw surfaces by removing fluid, thus help in rapid healing.

Caution: Drains should be avoided in a developing hematoma with an underlying major arterial anastomosis. (It's better to urgently address the cause of hemorrhage than to drain it.)

TYPES OF DRAIN

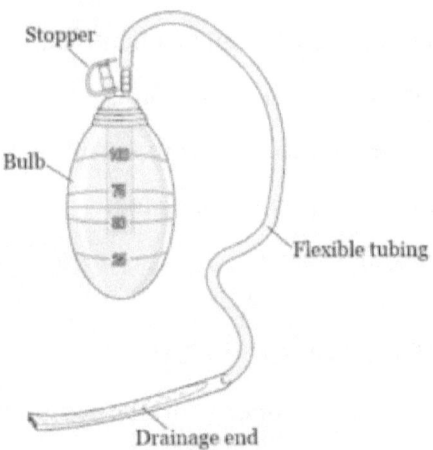

Stopper

Bulb

Flexible tubing

Drainage end

    i. Corrugated drain: Rubber drain or Transparent PVC drain: It drains by capillary action and gravity. It is technically easy to insert but it allows soakage of the dressing, necessitating dressing change.

   ii. Tube Drains:

      a. Nasogastric Tube, Foley's Catheter, Malecot's, Chest tube, Abdominal Tube drain.

      b. Penrose Drain

      c. Multiple perforated drain

   iii. Closed Suction Tube Drain: Jackson Pratt drain, Redivac Drain

   iv. Glove drain: Glove finger is used as a drain

   v. Wick Drain is a gauze drain. It may be used when other options are not readily available.

ADVANTAGES OF A TUBE DRAINS

   i. Draining effluent can be quantified.

   ii. It can be kept for longer time.

   iii. Chances of infection from outside are lessened.

   iv. Skin excoriation is prevented.

   v. Removal is easier.

CLASSIFICATION OF DRAINS

Based on usage and property, drains can be classified as follows:

   i. According to the Mechanism of Action: (a) Passive Drain (b) Active Drain

   ii. Nature: (a) Tube (b) Flat/Sheet

   iii. Disposition of Drain (a) Open (b) Closed

iv. **Location**: (a) Internal (b) External

v. **Property of Drain** (a) Inert (b) Irritant

vi. **Diagnostic v/s Therapeutic**

Open Drain

Open drains include corrugated rubber or plastic sheets and soak fluid in gauze pad dressing. PVC drain causes less tissue reaction. The risk of infection from outside is more than a closed drain.

Disadvantages: Retrograde infection & soiling of dressing necessitating frequent change.

Closed Drain

These include variety of tubes that drain into a collecting bag (closed from the environment). These include chest and abdominal drains. Often the closed drains are internally coated with silicone – an inert and slippery material that avoids the drain effluent from sticking inside the drain and clogging it.

Advantage: Since they are closed to the environment, chances of retrograde infection are less. They help to provide accurate fluid output measurement.

Facilitate radiographic studies, and protect the skin from irritants of discharge.

Disadvantages: Closed drains are vulnerable to obstruction due to: i) Adjoining tissue; ii) Ingrowth of organisms or tissue; iii) Drain effluent getting stuck in non-siliconized tubes.

Active Drains (Suction Drains)

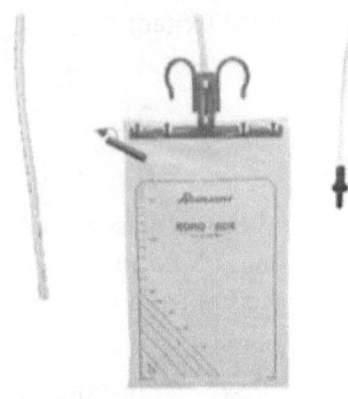

Tube drains that are aided by active suction, could be further reclassified into: Low continuous, Low intermittent or High suction based on the amount of suction pressure.

Advantage: They facilitate constant movement of thick exudates and necrotic material to the receptacle. Effluent can be measured. There is decreased risk of wound infection. No skin excoriation. However, regular evacuation of reservoir is often required.

Disadvantage: It may injure the adjacent tissues which may get sucked in. May not be safe to deploy the drain next to a bowel or vascular anastomosis. Suction may disrupt the anastomosis.

Passive Drains (Free Flow Drain)

These drains serve to evacuate fluid by the action of gravity and by the intra-cavitary pressure differentials. e.g: Intercostal and Abdominal tube drains.

Advantage: Since there is no active suction used, unlike active drains (which have suction) they can be safely used near bowel or vascular anastomosis.

Disadvantage: They are prone to get clogged due to thick exudate or slow moving necrotic material.

Diagnostic Drain

Drains may be used for diagnosis of complications eg. Biliary Fistula T-Tube Cholangiogram for CBD injury, retained gallstones in CBD (where a tubogram or a drainogram can be done in post-op period to detect retained gall stones).

Therapeutic Drain

Drains are used in various conditions, to promote escape of fluids already accumulated to relieve the symptoms such as:

    i. Tension pneumothorax or hydro-pneumothorax.

    ii. Abscess Drainage.

    iii. Seroma Drainage.

    iv. Acute urinary retention.

    v. Acute suppurative arthritis.

DUAL PURPOSE DRAIN (DIAGNOSTIC & THERAPEUTIC)

Pigtail Drain: These are special drains, whose one end curls up like the tail of a pig. They are used for percutaneous drainage of an abscess or a collection e.g: Liver abscess, post surgical abdominal collection & Pancreatic abscesses. i) These are useful in Unilocular collection/abscess; ii) Single, communicating; iii) Low viscous collection; iv) Drain route not transversing intra-abdominal organs or thorax.

Steps of Putting an Abdominal Drain

i. A drain should be placed always in the most dependent position and should be brought out through the shortest straight route.

ii. A skin stab incision is made with a 11-size blade away from the main wound.

iii. With the hand, kept as protective gear inside the wound, a Kelly clamp is inserted through the incision traversing the layers to abdominal wall.

iv. Drain tip is caught in Kelly's clamp and is pulled out through the tunnel.

v. Care should be taken to keep the tubing free from kinks, debris and clots so as to enhance free drainage.

vi. Finally, the drain position is secured with a skin suture and connected to an appropriate bag.

vii. Fixing of Drain: (Note: It is an important step of deployment of drain)

    a. Corrugated Drain – Simple loose loop suture of 02/0 Black silk and a safety pin.

    b. Tube & Suction Drain 02/0 block silk "Roman Sandal pattern of fixation" – with "Beading" in between ligature loops to avoid slippage & accidental removal.

CARE OF DRAIN

General Care

i. Skin around the drain should be kept dry at all times to prevent infection & irritation.

ii. Using universal precautions, drains should be dressed as indicated.

iii. Clots in the drains should be cleared to keep it patent.

iv. The drain reservoir should be emptied daily and a note should be made on the amount and its characteristics.

REMOVAL OF DRAIN

Generally, drains being foreign objects should be removed as soon as its intended purpose has been served. However general guidelines are:

i. Prophylactic drains are removed within 48 hours, or as soon as the drainage has subsided.

ii. Therapeutic drains are kept in its position until the drainage subsides. It is then gradually withdrawn each day 3–4cm/day and refixed. It allows closure of the drainage tract from its depth and prevents pocketing.

iii. Abdominal drains can be taken out when it discharges straw colored discharge of less than 25–30ml/day.

iv. Remove if it is blocked.

v. When it is a cause of an infection leading to sepsis.

COTTON GAUZE DRAIN

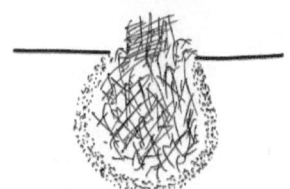

Gauze acts as a drain by capillary action of the gauze which absorbs the fluid. But once it fully soaked, it acts like a plug rather than a drain. So there is need to change at least once in 24 hrs.

WICKS

The wick is formed from gauze or threads of ligatures or suture material twisted together or bound loosely. When a wick is made of folded gauze, it swells upon soaking and may obstruct the tract. It becomes ineffective due to the soaking.

GLOVE RUBBER DRAIN

A strip of a glove, can be used to drain the superficial dead space. It is a poor drain and gets blocked easily, but is least irritant.

RED RUBBER CORRUGATED DRAIN (SHEET DRAIN)

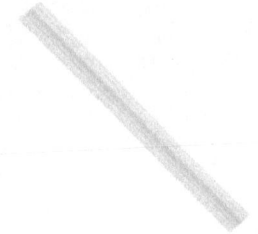

It is made up of red rubber which is available in the form of unsterile sheets, from which the strips of required length and breadth are cut and sterilized by autoclaving. Drainage of the fluid occurs along the grooves of the drain, so chances of blockage are less. If used for a prolonged period it results in sinus formation or pocket formation. It may be sucked into the wound when it is not fixed properly to the surface.

Currently portex drain is used instead of red rubber drain as it is less irritant than the red rubber.

Uses: These drains are used after a pyelolithotomy, in large abscess drainage, retropubic space and mastectomy.

TUBE DRAIN

A tube drain helps in collecting the fluid into a collection device.

Tube drains have to be bigger in size when draining blood or purulent material.

Catheters are also Tube Drains

Catheters (Red rubber catheter, Malecot's catheter and Foley's Catheter) are used when output is high eg. urine. Catheters can be used for draining of viscera like eg. cholecystostomy & caecostomy. They are also used for draining liver abscess, empyema thoracis & pyonephrosis.

PENROSE DRAIN

It is a hollow tube of latex rubber with a thin wall and can be made by cutting the finger stall of a surgical glove.

PORTEX DRAINAGE TUBE

They are made up of soft portex making them elastic and less irritant.

Uses: It has side holes and also at tip. A radio-opaque line along its length helps it to be located on xrays.

YEATES DRAIN

It is a sheet formed of parallel tubes of plastic material which tend to block often.

CIGARETTE DRAIN

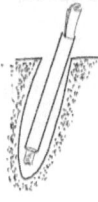

Penrose drain that has gauze within it is called a cigarette drain. Here the latex tube acts as conduit. The drainage comes out along it and not through the gauze. It can cause skin excoriation and ascending infection.

SHIRLEY DRAIN

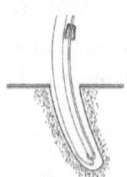

It has a side tube guarded by a bacterial filter so that the sterile air can be drawn down to the tip of the drain.

When suction is applied to the drain, the tissues are not sucked into the drain holes. Shirley drain is tube drain which is a double lumen drainage tube in which the side tube has multiple holes.

T-TUBE

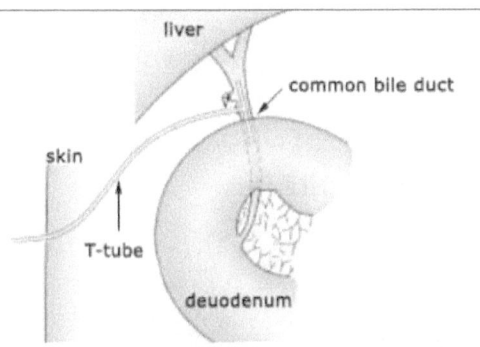

T-shaped tube is a long tube with another tube connected to it at right angle and it is presterilized (gamma rays or ethylene oxide). It is used to drain common bile duct after choledochotomy or choledochoenterostomy.

SUMP

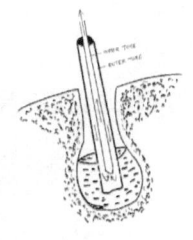

Sump drain is made up of two tubes, one in other. Outer tube has multiple holes, inner tube has a side holes and is connected to suction. When suction is applied, air is sucked in through the outer tube & out through the inner tube. Fluid collecting in the outer tube is sucked away. Since there is no suction on the outer tube, surrounding tissues are not drawn in it.

These drains are generally used to drain against the force of gravity. e.g. Drainage of pancreatic, duodenal, jejunal and ileal fistulae.

Advantages are: Output can be measured. Suction does not plug the drain.

Disadvantage is that it may erode the surrounding organs.

PLASTIC TUBE DRAIN

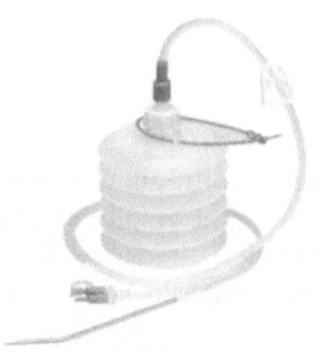

These may be made up of PVC or silastic and are connected to sterile containers. e.g. Negative Suction Tube Drain (**Redivac Suction Drain**): Most commonly used drains after major surgeries like eg. thyroid surgery, mastectomy, repair of incisional hernia and LN dissections etc. Plastic tube drain without suction are used following surgery on kidney ureter, urinary bladder etc.

INTELLIGENT DEPLOYMENT OF DRAINS

a. The foremost thing is to decide whether to drain or not to drain. If decided in favour of drainage then identify

   i. What to drain? (blood, pus, fluid, bile, feces etc.)

   ii. What volume of drainage is anticipated?

   iii. What kind of drain to be used (open, closed, free flow or suction drain)

   iv. Which is the most dependent area of the operated site where the fluid will collect?

b. Place the drain without kink or loop at the most dependent site for collection.

c. The drain should exit the skin surface, at the shortest distance from the site to be drained.

d. Open Drain (corrugated rubber or PVC) should not have tight exit from skin. The "skin incision" should be wide enough to facilitate, free flow of effluent.

e. Closed Drains (tube drains & suction drains) should have snug fitting skin exit, to avoid leakage of effluent and air.

Complications and their Prevention

Majority of the complications with drains are due to poor drain selection, placement and post-operative management.

i. **Infection:** Open Drains are in contact with the outside environment, thus breach the skin barrier leading to increase chances of hospital acquired infection. Strict aseptic & proper drain care.

ii. **Pain**

a. Tight fitting Tubes or Big diameter tubes.

b. Stiff and hard tubes/kinking of tubes.

iii. **Inefficient Drainage** occurs when a tube gets kinked, obstructed or diameter is small and fluid is thick. Poor placement is another important factor.

iv. **Tissue reaction:** Drains are foreign bodies and initiating significant tissue irritation. Use of non-irritant material such as silicone helps to ease the problem.

v. **Disintegration:** Drains should be secured firmly with the skin using non-absorbable suture. When kept for long, they can disintegrate and cause foreign body reaction.

vi. **Migration:** Drains can be sucked in prompt exploration of the wound and removal.

vii. **Drain entrapment:** Long term drain placement causes fibrous adhesions around it.

viii. **Bowel herniation:** Drain sites after removal if small should be left to close on its own, but when large, should be sutured with 1–2 sutures. Otherwise bowel herniation may occur.

Tips & Tricks

- Keep drains as minimal as possible, as short as possible and preferably use closed drains.

- Never place a drain in close or direct contact with an anastomosis to prevent leakage due to erosion.

- Drains can be occluded/obstructed by adjacent tissue, so beware of these.

- Remove drains at the earliest, as soon as they have served their purpose.

CATHETER

A catheter is a thin hollow, flexible tube often made of soft plastic or rubber material with both ends open.

The word catheter is derived from the ancient Greek word 'kathie´nai', which literally means "to thrust into" or "to send down". The earliest record of catheterization for treatment of urinary retention can be found in an ancient Egyptian Ebers papyrus around 1500 BC with the use oftrans-uretheral bronze tubes, reeds, straws and curled-up palm leaves. Almost 3000 years later, Ambroise Pare (1510–1590) devised a silver tube with a long gentle curve for easier insertion. Since then lot of development has taken place in the realm of catheters.

Types of Catheters

Based on Retention: i) Non Self- Retaining catheter (Ordinary catheter): Simple red rubber catheter, Condom catheter, Metallic catheter. ii) Self Retaining catheter: Foley's catheter, Malecot's catheter, Gibbon's catheter, De-Pezzer catheter

According to its Usage: i) Urethral and Supra-pubic; ii) Ureteric; iii) Endotracheal: suction catheter

According to its material: i) Metal; ii) Gum elastic; iii) Rubber; iv) Plastic; v) Silicone.

Types of Catherisation

i. **Indwelling Catheterization:** When the catheter is left behind in the urinary bladder and remains so, it is called an indwelling catherization. eg: Foley's catherization of urinary bladder, insertion of pig-tail catheter in liver abscess.

ii. **Intermittent Catheterization:** When catheterization is done once and the catheter is removed after drainage of urine. Intermittent self catheterization is a long term domicile treatment of neurogenic bladder.

Simple Red Rubber Catheter

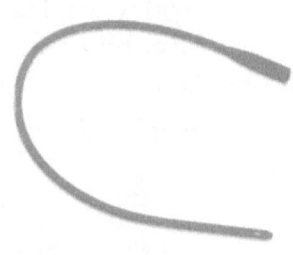

These non self retaining red tubes, are stiffer than Foley's catheter, and are made of India rubber. The tip is round and blunt whistle tip. It is used in acute urinary retention. They are available in sizes 3–12 and are each 37.5cm long. However, they are not used in routine practice these days.

Metallic Catheter

They are not used in routine practice these days.

Self-Retaining Malecot's Catheter

Made up of latex (earlier ones were made of red rubber), malecot tubes have wings (flower like appearance)

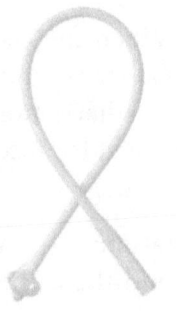

which promote drainage and retention of the tube in its intended place. It is used for drainage of Empyema of chest, gallbladder, bladder & pyonephrosis of kidney. They are not much in practice these days due to availability of modern tubes and drains made of silicon.

Foley's Catheter

In 1929, Dr Frederic Foley designed the modern balloon-based self-retaining catheter.

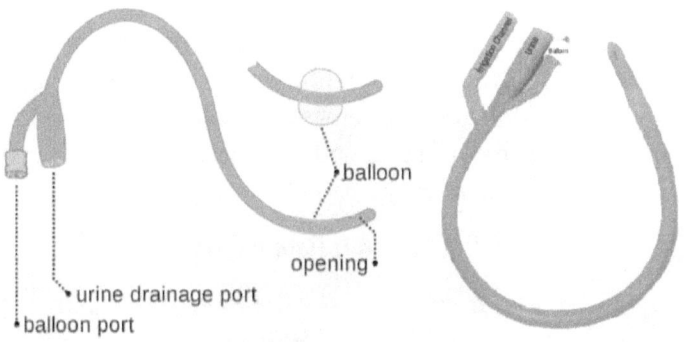

It has two channels, one for the drainage of urine and the second for balloon inflation to retain the catheter within the bladder. It could be triple lumen which is used during TUR for irrigation. The smooth rounded tip of the catheter extends beyond the balloon and one or more eye-holes are adjacent to the blunt and smooth tip to allow urine to drain. The balloon channel has a valve incorporated near the end so that fluid can be injected to inflate the balloon.

Sizes: They are available in various sizes in French scale. (1F= 0.33mm diameter), Smaller sizes are used in children.

Latex catheters coated with hydrogel – last 12 weeks.

Polytetrafluoroethylene (PTFE) or Teflon® – these can be used for up to 28 days;

Silicone elastomer is a biologically inert nonstickey material and is coated on a latex core.

100% silicone – Can last for 12 weeks and are hypoallergenic

Balloon

After a catheter has been successfully inserted, usually up to the hilt, the balloon should not be inflated until urine starts draining, to ensure correct position. The balloon must be inflated with sterile water (10–30ml) which is mentioned on the catheter itself.

Do not use the following to inflate balloons:

i. Air – can result in the balloon floating in the bladder and thus poor drainage.

ii. Non-sterile water – may contain impurities and bacteria that can enter the bladder through diffusion or if balloon ruptures.

iii. Saline – saline can crystallize and can deposit in the inflating channel or the balloon itself, which can cause problems when deflating the balloon to take the catheter out.

PRINCIPAL REASONS FOR CATHERIZATION OF URINARY BLADDER

i. **Drainage:**

- Acute and chronic urinary retention, neurogenic bladder, trauma

- Post operative, TURB, urinary incontinence.

ii. **Monitor:** Monitor fluid balance - usually in critically ill patients

   iii. **Instillation:** Bladder instillations of drugs like BCG and chemotherapeutic agents in Ca. Bladder.

   iv. Obtaining a **urine sample**.

   v. **Investigation:** Radiological evaluation of lower urinary tract – cystogram/urethrogram.

   vi. For accurate measurements of urinary output

  vii. Palliative care.

 viii. Urodynamics

CARE OF CATHETERS

- Cleanse the urethral area (where the catheter exits the body) and the catheter itself.

- Make sure that urine is flowing from the catheter into the urine collection bag and the tube is not twisted or kinked.

- The urine collection bag should be kept below the level of the urinary bladder.

- Check for inflammation or signs of infection in the area around the catheter at tip of urethra.

COMPLICATIONS OF FOLEY'S CATHERIZATION

Immediate (Within 2 hrs)

- Urethral Injury
  - i. Directly by the catheter in difficult catheterization

ii. Inflating balloon before insuring correct catheterplacement in the Bladder. False Passage – by injury to the urethral wall during insertion.

iii. Bacteraemia & ascending infection.

- Paraphimosis due to failure to return foreskin to normal position following catheter insertion.

Late Complications

i. Urethral Strictures following damage to the urethra.

ii. Bladder Stone formation on a piece of ruptured balloon.

iii. Ascending Urinary tract infections

iv. Impacted urinary catheter.

Chapter 3

SUTURES AND NEEDLES

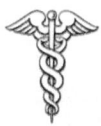

Pradeep Garg

Suture materials are used to **close all types of wounds** whether external or internal. The ideal suture should allow the **healing tissue** to recover adequately **to keep the wound closed** together once sutures are **removed or absorbed**.

The time it takes for a tissue to no longer require support from sutures will vary depending on tissue type:

Days: Muscle, subcutaneous tissue or skin

Weeks to Months: Fascia or tendon

Months to Never: Vascular prosthesis

The following are required for suture closure of a wound:

- Suture material

- Needle

- Needle holder

The suture material is a foreign body to human tissues and provokes a foreign-body tissue reaction. During wound closure, a sterile arena and careful aseptic technique are essential to minimize the risk of wound infection.

Surgical needles are produced from stainless steel alloys, which have excellent resistance to corrosion. All true stainless steels contain a minimum of 12% chromium, which allows a thin, protective surface layer of chromium oxide to form when the steel is exposed to oxygen. Wound closure and healing are affected by the initial tissue injury caused by needle penetration and subsequent suture passage. Proper needle selection, surface characteristics of the suture (e.g., coefficient of friction), and suture-coating materials used for wound closure are very important factors which affect wound healing.

At present, no single available suture material has all ideal characteristics. Suture characteristics vary according to different areas of the body.

All sutures must possess the following fundamental and essential characteristics:

- Sterility

- Uniform diameter and size

- Ease of handling and knot security

- Uniform tensile strength

- Freedom from irritants or impurities that could cause tissue reaction

Besides these, there are various other characteristics of suture material that are described in the following terms:

- Absorbent - Progressive loss of mass or volume of suture material; this does not correlate with initial tensile strength

- Breaking strength - Limit of tensile strength at which suture failure occurs

- Capillarity - Extent to which absorbed fluid is transferred along the suture

- Elasticity - Measure of the ability of the material to regain its original form and length after deformation

- Fluid absorption - Ability to soak up fluid after immersion

- Knot-pull tensile strength - Breaking strength of knotted suture material (10–40% weaker after deformation by knot placement)

- Knot strength - Amount of force necessary to cause a knot to slip (this is related to the coefficient of static friction and plasticity of a given material)

- Memory - Inherent capability of suture to return to or maintain its original gross shape (this is related to elasticity, plasticity, and diameter)

- Nonabsorbable - Surgical suture material that is relatively unaffected by the biologic activities of the body tissues and is therefore permanent, unless removed

- Plasticity - Measure of the ability to deform without breaking and to maintain a new form after relief from the deforming force

- Pliability - Ease of handling of suture material; ability to adjust knot tension and to secure knots (this is related to suture material, filament type and diameter)

- Straight-pull tensile strength - Linear breaking strength of suture material

- Suture pullout value - Application of force to a loop of suture located where tissue failure occurs, which measures the strength of a particular tissue; this varies according to anatomic site and histologic composition (fat, 0.2 kg; muscle, 1.27 kg; skin, 1.82 kg; fascia, 3.77 kg)

- Tensile strength - Measure of the ability of a material or tissue to resist deformation and breakage

- Wound breaking strength - Limit of tensile strength of a healing wound at which separation of the wound edges occurs

Suture size refers to the diameter of the suture strand and is denoted by means of zeroes. The more zeroes characterizing a bigger suture size, the smaller, the resultant strand diameter (e.g., 4–0 or 0000 is *bigger in diameter* than 5–0 or 00000). The smaller the suture, the lesser the tensile strength of the strand.

SUTURE CLASSIFICATION

Sutures may be classified in terms of their origin, their structure, and their absorbability. Both absorbable and non-absorbent surgical sutures can be made from either natural or synthetic polymers.

ABSORBABLE SUTURE MATERIALS

These sutures are absorbed by the body and do not require removal. These sutures are available as braided and monofilament.

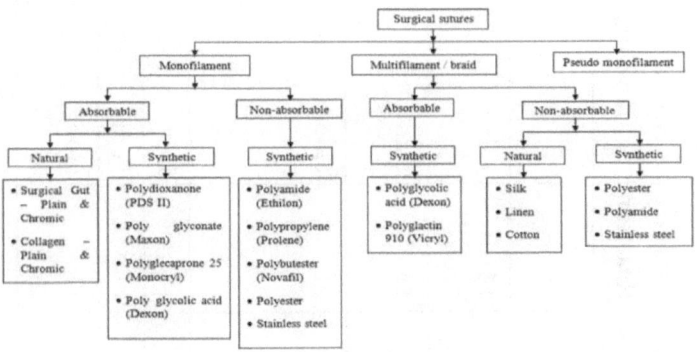

Brand Name	Material	Tensile Strength	Tissue Reaction	Behavior & Handling	Knot Quality	Absorption of Suture
1. COLLAGEN (Plain/Chromic)	Beef Tendon	Poor	+2	Fair	Poor	1 to 2 weeks
2. SURGICAL GUT (plain)	Animal collagen	Poor	+4	Fair	Poor	1 to 2 weeks
3. SURGICAL GUT (chromic)	Animal collagens	Poor	+3	Fair	Fair	1 to 2 weeks
4. VICRYL	Polyglactin 910 coated polyglactin 370 & calcium sterate	Good	+1	Good	Fair	3 months
5. DEXON "S"	Polyglycolic	Good	+1	Fair	Good	3 months
6. PDS	Polydioxanone	Good	+1	Poor	Poor	6 months
7. MONOCRYL	Polyglicaprone 25	Fair	+1	Good	Good	3 months

Tensile Strength:

- POOR = absorbed and 0% strength by 3 weeks
- GOOD = 50% strength remains by 3 weeks
- FAIR = 20% strength remains by 3 weeks

*Tissue Reaction = tendency to cause inflammation + low, +4 high

*Behaviour and Handling = easy to use suture

*Knot quality = tendency to stay

NON-ABSORBABLE SUTURES

These sutures are not absorbed by body and require removal. Silk is only braided and rest is monofilament.

Brand Name	Material	Behavior & Handling	Knot Quality	Tissue Reaction
Silk	Silk	Good	Fair	+4
Mersilene	Polyester	Good	Good	+2
Dacron	Polyester	Good	Good	+2
Ethibond	Polyester	Good	Good	+2
Stainless Steel	Stainless Steel	Poor	Good	+1
Ethilon	Polyamide (Nylon)	Fair	Fair	+2
Dermalon	Polyamide (Nylon)	Poor	Poor	+2
Surgamid	Polyamide (Nylon)	Poor	Poor	+2

Brand Name	Material	Behavior & Handling	Knot Quality	Tissue Reaction
Nurolon	Polyamide (Nylon)	Good	Fair	+2
Prolene	Polyolefin (Polypropylene)	Poor	Poor	+1

*Tissue Reaction = tendency to cause inflammation, + low, +4 high

*Behaviour & Handling = easy to use suture

*Knot quality = tendency to stay

The lower the suture size number, the larger (thicker) the diameter and the higher (greater, stronger) the tensile strength.

The higher the suture size number, the smaller (thinner) the diameter and the lower (less, weaker) the tensile strength.

Choose suture according to required site

Site	Skin layers (suture size)	Sutures	Deep layers (suture size)	Sutures
Scalp	Silk, Nylon, polypropylene or staples	3–0, 4–0	2–0 to 4–0	Absorbable, Chromic catgut or Polyglactin 910

Site	Skin layers (suture size)	Sutures	Deep layers (suture size)	Sutures
Face	Silk, Nylon, Polypropylene, Plain gut	5–0 to 6–0	3–0 to 5–0	-do-
Neck	Silk, Nylon, Polypropylene, Plain gut	4–0 to 5–0	2–0 to 4–0	-do-
Trunk	Silk, Nylon, Polypropylene or staples	2–0 to 4–0	2–0 to 3–0	-do-
Limbs	Silk, Nylon, Polypropylene or staples	3–0 to 5–0	2–0 to 4–0	-do-
Hands and Feet	Silk, Nylon, Polypropylene or staples	4–0 to 5–0	3–0 to 5–0	-do-
Soles of Feet	Silk, Nylon, Polypropylene or staples	2–0 to 4–0	2–0 to 4–0	-do-

NATURAL VS SYNTHETIC

Natural sutures can be made of collagen from mammalian intestines or from synthetic collagen (polymers). Tissue reaction and suture antigenicity lead to inflammatory reactions, especially with natural materials. Synthetic sutures are made of artificial polymers.

MONOFILAMENT VS MULTIFILAMENT

Monofilament suture material is made of a single strand; this structure is relatively more resistant to harboring microorganisms. It also exhibits less resistance to passage through tissue than multifilament suture does. However, great care must be taken in handling and tying a monofilament suture, because crushing or crimping of the suture can nick or weaken it and lead to undesirable and premature suture failure.

Multifilament suture material is composed of several filaments twisted or braided together. It generally has greater tensile strength and better pliability and flexibility than monofilament suture material, and it handles and ties well. However, because multifilament materials have increased capillarity, the increased absorption of fluid may facilitate the introduction of pathogens which increases the risk for wound infection and dehiscence.

NEEDLE QUALITIES

The ideal surgical needle would have the following features:

1. High-quality stainless steel

2. Smallest possible diameter

3. Cause minimal tissue trauma

4. Sterile and corrosion-resistant

Various Features of Working of Needle:

- Strength - Resistance to twist during repeated passes through tissue

- Ductility - Resistance (of a needle) to breaking due to bending

- Sharpness - The capability of the needle to pierce tissue

- Clamping moment - Stability of a needle in a needle holder due to interaction of the needle body with the jaws of the needle holder

NEEDLE CONSTRUCTION

A surgical needle has three sections: the point, the body, and the swage (see the image below). The point is the sharpest portion and is used to penetrate the tissue. The body represents the midportion of the needle. The swage is the thickest portion of the needle and the portion to which the suture material is attached.

Point

The point portion of the needle extends from the tip to the maximum cross-section of the body. Point types include the following (see the image below):

- Cutting needles (conventional, reverse, or side [spatula])

- Taper-point (round) needles

- Bevelled conventional cutting-edge needles

- Blunt-point needles

Sharpness is due to the cutting edges. A cutting needle has two opposing cutting edges (the point is usually triangular). Cutting needle is intended to pierce thick tissues and is ideal for skin sutures. Conventional cutting needles have three cutting edges (a triangular cross-section that changes to a flattened body). The third cutting edge is on the inner, concave curvature (surface-seeking).

In reverse-cutting needles, the third cutting edge is on the outer convex curvature of the needle. These needles are stronger than conventional cutting needles. They are created to pierce skin, tendon sheaths, or oral mucosa. Reverse-cutting needles are also beneficial in cosmetic and ophthalmic surgery, causing minimal trauma.

Side-cutting (spatula) needles are flat on the top and bottom surfaces to reduce tissue injury. These needles allow maximum ease of penetration and were created for ophthalmic procedures.

Taper-point (round) needles pierce and pass through tissues by stretching without cutting. The sharpness is determined by the taper ratio (8-12:1) and the tip angle (20-35°). The needle is sharper if it has a higher taper ratio and a lower tip angle. The taper-point needle is used for easily penetrated tissues.

A bevelled conventional cutting needle is superior to other conventional cutting needles. It is composed of a unique stainless steel, ASTM 45500, that is heat-treated after the curving process to enhance its resistance to bending. The angle of presentation of the cutting edge is decreased to enhance sharpness. This beveled conventional cutting needle is recommended for closure of lacerations.

Blunt point needles dissect friable tissue rather than cut it. The points are rounded and blunt, ideal for suturing the soft organs like liver and kidneys. Thus, there is minimum injury to friable tissues.

Body

Needle body types include the following:

- Straight body
- Half-curved ski body
- Curved body
- Compound curved body

The body part of the needle includes most of the needle length and is vital for interaction with the needle holder and the ability to deliver piercing force to the needle point. So, needle diameter and radius, body geometry, and stainless-steel alloy are very essential.

The straight-body needle is used to suture easily accessible tissue that can be manipulated directly by hand. It is also used in microsurgery for nerve and vessel repair.

The half-curved ski needle is rarely used in skin closure, because of its handling features. The straight portion of the body does not follow the curved point, resulting in an enlarged curved point that makes the needle difficult to handle.

The curved needle needs less space than a straight needle to pass through tissue. The semicircular path is the optimal course for sutures through tissue and provides an even distribution of tension. Body curvature commonly follows a 0.25-in., 0.375-in., 0.5-in., or 0.625-in. circle. The 0.375-in. circle is used most commonly for skin closure; the 0.5-in. circle was designed for confined spaces, and better tissue manipulation.

Swage

The suture attachment end creates a single, continuous unit of suture and needle, known as the swage. The swage is created to permit easy passage of the needle and suture material through tissue.

- Channel swage

- Drill swage

- Non-swaged

Several disadvantages are associated with the use of a non-swaged needle. Passage of a double strand of suture through tissue leads to more tissue trauma.

Coating

The needle may be coated with silicone to permit easier tissue passage without trauma.

NEEDLE–NEEDLE HOLDER INTERACTION

The jaws of the needle holder must be appropriate to the needle size to hold it steadily and prevent rocking, turning, and rotation of the needle, interaction between needle holder and suture needle.

The needle-holder handle must be appropriate for the required depth of suture placement. The difference between the length of the handle and the jaw creates a mechanical advantage for exerting force through the needle point (Lever Action).

The needle-holder squeezing moment is the force applied to a suture needle by a needle holder. Technically speaking, the needle-holder holding/squeezing moment must be less than the surgical yield of the needle, or the needle will bend and ultimately may break. A bent needle takes a relatively traumatic path through soft tissue and may cause increased soft-tissue injury.

Repetitive injury by the needle holder also may cause the needle to break. If the broken portion of the needle is not identified and retrieved immediately, surgery may be delayed in an effort to find it. The need for intraoperative radiology and other potential difficulties may ensue.

This damage to the suture can be prevented by mechanically grinding the outer edges of the smooth tungsten carbide inserts so as to achieve a rounded edge.

Take Home Message

Always use proper size of suture along with proper size and nature of Needle for proper wound suturing and subsequent healing.

REFERENCES

1. "Suture Materials - Classification - Surgical Needles - TeachMeSurgery"

2. "Types of Sutures". Dolphin Sutures. Retrieved 2014-01-07.

3. Surgical Needle Guide from Novartis. Copyright 2005.

4. ETHICON Products (20 December 2002). "ETHICON Receives FDA Clearance to Market VICRYL* Plus, First Ever Antibacterial Suture". PRNewswire. Retrieved 25 January 2016.

5. Daoud, FC; Edmiston CE, Jr; Leaper, D (June 2014). "Meta-analysis of prevention of surgical site infections following incision closure with triclosan-coated sutures: robustness to new evidence". Surgical Infections. **15** (3):16581. doi:10.1089/ sur.2013.177. PMC 4063374. PMID 24738988.

Chapter 4

ANTIBOITICS SELECTION DURING EMERGENCY

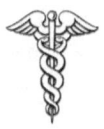

Antibiotics are used to treat infections in body. After culture and sensitivity, specific antibiotics are given. Unnecessarily use of antibiotics increases the risk of bacteria developing resistance to antibiotics. Antibiotic resistance is a growing problem across the world. Classification of antibiotics depends upon their mechanism of action, chemical structure, or spectrum of activity. Antibiotics are static or bactericidal in function. [1] They effect the bacterial cell wall (penicillins and cephalosporins) or the cell membrane (polymyxins), or obstruct the essential bacterial enzymes (rifamycins, lipiarmycins, quinolones, and sulfonamides) to have bactericidal activities. Antibiotics which act through protein synthesis (macrolides, lincosamides and tetracyclines) are usually bacteriostatic (with the exception of bactericidal aminoglycosides).[2] Further classification is based on killing range i.e. spectrum.

"Narrow-spectrum means antibiotics for Gram-negative or Gram-positive bacteria, whereas broad-spectrum antibiotics influence a wide range of bacteria.[3,4]

ANTIBIOTICS DOSES AND TOXICITIES

Agent	Usual Adult Doses	Adverse Effects
1-Penicillins Beta-Lactamase Susceptible, Non antipseudomonal Penicillins Penicillin G	IV low dose: 600.000-1200,000 U/d IV high dose: 4M U load, then 1M U q1h	Hypersensitivity: drug fever, rash Anaphylactic reactions (approx.1in10,000) Blood positive Coombs, Hemolytic anemia, Cytopenia, nephrotoxicity Seizures, phlebitis at IV site

Agent	Usual Adult Doses	Adverse Effects
Benzathine penicillin	IM:600,000-1200,000 U qid IV 1-3 g q4-6h	Not for IV use same with penicillin G, plus local reaction at injection site Rash, fever, low WBC, high SGOT, anaphylactic reaction, Interstitial nephritis, convulsions (with excessive rapid infusion)
Ampicillin	IV 2-4 g q4-6h	Similar to other penicillin Similar to Ampicillin alone
Beta-Lactamase Susceptible,	IV 3.1 g q4-6h	Similar to Ampicillin alone
Antipseudomonal Penicillins-	IV 1.5 g q6h	Similar to Piperacillin alone

Agent	Usual Adult Doses	Adverse Effects
Piperacillin	IV 3.375 g q4-6h	
Combination Beta-Lactamase Inhibitors & Beta-Lactam Agents *Ticarcillin-clavulanic acid *Ampicillin-sulbactum *Pipercillin-tazobactum	Moderate infection: IV/IM 1 g q4h Severe infection: IV: 2 g q4h For: pseudomonas; use q4h regimen	Phlebitis, rash, drug fever, eosinophilia, hemolytic anemia, neutropenia, interstitial nephritis, nausea, diarrhea, elevated SGOT
Beta-lactamase Resistant Penicillin *Nafcillin	Moderate infection: IV/IM: 1g q4h Severe infection: IV: 2 g q4h IV/IM: 0.5-3 g q6-8h	Similar to nafcillin, neutropenia less frequent Rash, elevated SGOT, elevated alkaline phosphatase, phlebitis, positive Coombs Rash

Agent	Usual Adult Doses	Adverse Effects
*Oxacillin	IV/IM: 2 g q12h	phlebitis, rash, esinophilia, positive Coombs, neutropenia
2-CEPHALOSPORIN/ CEPHAMYCINS/ CARBACEPHEM	Moderate infection: IV/ IM 1 g q8-12h	do- and mildly elevated BUN, Falsely elevated serum creatinine
	Life-threatening infection: IV/IM: 2 g q4h IV/IM: 1-2 g q4-6h	-do- and diarrhea -do- Most common adverse reactions: gastrointestinal (nausea, vomiting, diarrhea), and allergic reactions (anaphylaxis, urticaria, skin rash). (6)
*Cefazolin	IV/IM: 0.5-2 g q8-12h	do- and elevated LDH, bilirubin, nausea, diarrhea

Agent	Usual Adult Doses	Adverse Effects
*Cefepime	IV/IM: 0.5-2 g q12-24h	Hypersensitivity: rash, pruritis, eosinophilia, positivecooms, neutropenia, oliguria, elevated SGOT, SGPT, alkaline phosphatase, confusion, seizures, myoclonus, nausea, vomiting, diarrhea, pseudomembranous colitis, high incidence of neurological side effects in elderly patients with poor renal function, with CV disease, or seizure disorder
* Cefotaxime	IV/IM: 0.75-1.5 g q8h	
*Cefoxitin	IV: 1-2 g q8h	
*Ceftazidime	IV : 1 g q24h	
*Ceftriaxone	IV: 0.5-1 g q6-8h	
*Cefuroxime	IV: 0.75 to 1.5 grams 8hrly	

Agent	Usual Adult Doses	Adverse Effects
3.CARBAPENEMS--- *Meropenem	Moderately severe infection: IV: 1 g q8h Life-threatening infection: IV: 2 g q6h	skin rash, constipation, Diarrhoea, Headache, Nausea , Vomiting
Ertapenem	IV: 1.5 mg/kg/d divided q8h	Similar to meropenem Similar to meropenem
*Imipenemcilastatin	IV:3-5mg/kg/ddividedq8h	
4. MONOBACTAMS--- *Aztreonam	IV:3-5mg/kg/d divided q8h IM: 0.5-2 g/d	Phlebitis, Hypersensitivity, elevated SGOT, Diarrhea, nausea, vomiting, seizures. It is sodium free drug

Agent	Usual Adult Doses	Adverse Effects
5. AMINOGLYCOSIDES and RELATEDANTIBIOTICS- *Amikacin	 IV: 500mg 8-12hly	Nephrotoxicity (proteinuria, elevated BUN), Ototoxicity, eosinophilia, arthralgia, fever, skin rash, probable neuromuscular blockade
		Same as above
*Gentamicin	IV: 3-5mg/kg/ day divided every 8hrly	
*Tobramycin	IV: 5mg/kg/day in 3-4 divided doses	same as above
6.FLUOROQUINOLONES- *Ciprofloxacin	IV: 400mg 12hrly	Nausea, vomiting, diarrhea, abdominal pain, Headache, insomnia, nightmare, toxic psychosis, confusion, seizures, rash, angioedema, elevated SGOT, alkaline phosphatase, WBC, creatinine same as above

Agent	Usual Adult Doses	Adverse Effects
*Gatifloxacin	IV: 400 mg/12hrly	same as above
*Levofloxacin	IV: 500 mg 12hrly	same as above
*Ofloxacin	IV: 400 mg 12hrly	same as above
*Moxifloxacin	400 mg OD daily	
7.MACROLIDES— *Azithromycin	500 mg orally 1st day, 250 mgs 2-5 days	Nausea, diarrhea, abdominal pain,
8. GLYCOPEPTIDES- *Clindamycin	600.1200 mg/day in 2,3 or 4 equal doses	Diarrhea, pseudomembranous colitis with toxic megacolon, rash, neutropenia, esinophilia, Nausea, vomiting, abdominal cramps, diarrhea,
*Erythromycin	500 mg tablet every 12 hours	phlebitis, fever, rash, Ototoxicity, neutropenia, esinophilia,

Agent	Usual Adult Doses	Adverse Effects
*Vancomycin	1 gm every 12 hours	anaphylactoid reactions, Red man syndrome- (flushing over upper chest)
9.CHALORAMPHENICOL-		Rarely used as it causes aplasia, aplastic anemia, fever, rash, anaphylactoid reaction, optic atrophy or neuropathy, digital paresthesia.

PROPHYLACTIC ANTIBIOTICS

Antibiotic is infused during the 1-hour period prior to surgery for prophylactic purpose. Quinolones and vancomycin are given 2 hours prior to surgery. For prolonged surgery or when there is extensive blood loss, more doses are given at intervals 1-2 times the half-life of drug. Postoperative antibiotics are given for major surgeries. In case of perforated viscous antibiotics are given for 8-10 days in post-operative period.

Procedures	Prophylactic Drug/Drugs	Drug Regime
Herniorraphy	None	
Mastectomy	None	

Procedures	Prophylactic Drug/Drugs	Drug Regime
Cholecystectomy	None or	
	Cefazolin or	1-2 g IV preoperatively +/- q12hx 1-3 d
	Clindamycin +	600mg IV preoperatively (+/- q8h x
		24 h
	gentamicin	1.5mg/kg IV preoperatively (+/- q8h x 24 h
Appendectomy	Cefoxitin or	2 g IV preoperatively (+/_q6h x 3 doses if nonperforated and 3-5 days if perforated)
	Cefazolin + metronidazole	-do-
		500 mg IV preoperatively once if nonperforated and q8h x 3-5 d if perforated
	Alternatively- Ciprofloxacin +	400 mg preoperatively q6h x 3 doses if nonperforated, or for 3-5 d if perforated
	clindamycin	900 mg IV preoperatively once if nonperforated or preoperatively and q8h IV if perforated

Procedures	Prophylactic Drug/Drugs	Drug Regime
Gastrectomy	Cefazolin or Gentamicin + clindamycin or Ciprofloxacin	1 g IV preoperatively if high risk 120 mg IV preoperatively 600 mg IV preoperatively 400 mg IV preoperatively
colon Surgery	Oral (alone or with IV) Neomycin+ Erythromycin+ laxative IV Cefoxitin or Cefazolin+ Metronidazole Clindamycin + gentamicin or Ciprofloxacin	1 g PO of each antibiotic at 1 PM, 2 PM, 11PM preoperatively; 4L polyethylene glycol electrolyte solution PO over 2h at 10 AM preoperatively 1-2 g IV preoperatively (+_ q4h x3 1-2 g IV preoperatively plus 0.5-1.0 g IV 600mg IV x 3 1.5mg/kg IV x 1 400 mg IV x 1

Procedures	Prophylactic Drug/Drugs	Drug Regime
Penetrating Abdominal wound trauma	Cefoxitin	2 g IV upon hospital admission and 2 g IV q6h x 2-5 d if perforation found
Ruptured Viscus	Cefoxitin + gentamicin or Clindamycin + gentamicin	2 g IV pre-op 1 g IV q8h x >_ 5 d 1.5 mg/kg IV q8h x >_ 5 d 900 mg IV q8h x >_ 5 d 1.5 mg/kg IV q8h x >_ 5d
Prostatectomy	None Ciprofloxacin	400 mg if organism present

Wound Infections		Antibiotics
Slightly Infected Wound due to surgical trauma – **Mild or moderate** no sepsis (No viscous/gynae surgery)	Common pathogens	Bactrim DS twice daily orally OR Cephalexin 500mg 4 times daily orally OR Amoxyclav 625mg three times a day OR 1000mg twice a day OR Doxycycline 100mg twice daily OR Clindamycin 300mg to 450mg four times a day
Slightly Infected Wound due to surgical trauma – **severe infection** but no sepsis (No viscous/gynae surgery)		Piperacillin-tazobactam 3.375 grams IV every 6 hours **OR**

Wound Infections		Antibiotics
Wound infection + **sepsis**. (No viscous/ Gynae surgery)	Common Pathogens	Ampicillin – Tazobactum-1.5-3 gm 6hrly OR Piperacillin-tazobactam 3.375 grams IV every 6 hours **OR** Cefazolin 1 gram IV every 8 hours.
Post-op wound (surgery involving viscous/gynae surgery)	Common Pathogens + Anaerobes	Piperacillin-tazobactam 3.375 grams IV every 6 hours OR Ampicillin-sulbactam 1.5-3g ivpb q6h OR Cefataxime 1-2gms 8hrly Or Ceftrixone 1-2 gm 4hrly Plus Metronidazole 500mg 6-8hrly

Wound Infections		Antibiotics
		Imipenem 500mg – 1gm 6hrly

REFERENCES

1. Calderon CB, Sabundayo BP (2007). Antimicrobial Classifications: Drugs for Bugs. In Schwalbe R, Steele-Moore L, Goodwin AC. Antimicrobial Susceptibility Testing Protocols. CRC Press. Taylor & Frances group. ISBN 978-0-8247-4100-6

2. Finberg RW, Moellering RC, Tally FP; et al. (November 2004). "The importance of bactericidal drugs: future directions in infectious disease". Clin. Infect. Dis. **39** (9): 1314–20. doi:10.1086/425009. PMID 15494908.

3. Cunha BA. Antibiotic Essentials 2009. Jones & Bartlett Learning, ISBN 978-0-7637-7219-2 p. 180, for example.

4. Srivastava A, Talaue M, Liu S, Degen D, Ebright RY, Sineva E, Chakraborty A, Druzhinin SY, Chatterjee S, Mukhopadhyay J, Ebright YW, Zozula A, Shen J, Sengupta 5.S, Niedfeldt RR, Xin C, Kaneko T, Irschik H, Jansen R, Donadio S, Connell N, Ebright RH (2011). "New target for inhibition of bacterial RNA polymerase: 'switch region'". Curr.Opin.Microbiol.14 (5):532-43. doi:10.1016/j.mib.2011.07.030. PMC 3196380. PMID 21862392.

Chapter 5

FLUID AND ELECTROLYTES

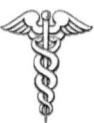

MK Garg

Electrolytes (minerals) have an electric charge in our body. Sodium, calcium, potassium, chlorine, phosphate and magnesium are all electrolytes and are present in body fluids and urine. We get them from the foods and the fluids we consume and they are responsible for muscle action. Medicines, vomiting, diarrhea, sweating or kidney problems can affect the level of electrolytes.

60% of body weight is fluid

Total Body Water=Weight in Kg. x 0.60 e.g.(70 kg x 0.60 = 4 2 litres)

2/3 is intracellular (28 litres-intracellular)

1/3 is extra cellular (14 litres-extra cellular)

So, if we give 3 litres of crystalloids, then 1litre of intravascular volume will be replaced.

Intravascular Volume = Plasma + Blood Cells

Weight in Kg. x 0.07 (70 x 0.07) = 4.9 litres

ESTIMATION OF MAINTENANCE FLUIDS

(Various formulae)

For Adults:-

1. 1.5 x body weight/hour e.g. 1.5 x 7 0 kg = 105 ml/ hour

2. 60 ml per hour for 1st 20 kg + 1 ml/kg/hour for rest of body weight

   e.g. 70 kg weight:- 60 + 50 = 110 ml/hour

3. Rule- 4-2-1

   • 4 ml/hour/kg body weight for the first 10 kg body weight (Max 40 ml)

   • 2 ml/hour X kg body weight for next 10 kgs body weight (Max 20 ml)

   • 1 ml/hour for each remaining body weight. e.g.-

   For 70 kg body weight :- 40 + 20 + 50 =110 ml/ hour

Types of Fluids

Dextrose 5%

Dextrose Saline

Normal Saline=154 mEq/L (Na + and 154mEq Chloride (cl)

½ Saline = 77 mEq/L (Na + and 77 mEq Chloride (cl)

Ringer Lactate–it contains-

130 mEq/L Na +

110 mEq/L Chloride (cl)

28 mEq/L lactate

4 mEq/L k +

1.3 mEq/L calcium

Isolyte-Gastric (G)

Isolyte Maintenance (M)

Isolyte Paediatrics (P)

Ideal Fluids for Diabetics Patients

Fructose

Ringer Lactate

Normal Saline

Ringer Lactate is also a classic fluid of choice for resuscitation.

For Renal Failure – Normal Saline is the fluid of choice.

For Neurosurgery – Ringer Lactate is the fluid of choice.

For Cardiac and Lung surgery – Albumin (25 g) is osmotically equivalent to 500 c.c. of normal saline, so, it's a good choice for cardiac surgery.

Normal requirement of Salt in a body per day is 5 gms – 600 of Normal Saline.

CVP Line is important to determine over/under hydration of body.

URINE OUTPUT is important to know hydration of patient.

Normal - 1–2 ml/minute.

Blood Urea estimation is the most sensitive index of the degree of depletion and efficiency of replacement.

The optimal Basal Intake of fluids per day is 2–3 litres.

For 24–48 hours after major surgery, sodium and water are retained by the body and urine output also decreases. So, in winter, the fluid requirement is only 2 litres/day. In summer it is up to 3 litres/day.

Rate of administration of fluid is —Required Fluid per day in litres x 11

For instance, if 2 litres/day is required then it drops per minute = 2 x11 = 22 drops per minute.

Amount of fluid to be given in hrs/4= number of macro drops per minute.

Orally about 100 ml is given per hour.

Input Output Chart is very important.

ACIDOSIS – (DECREASED ALKALI RESERVE IN BODY)

Causes

- Prolonged Diarrhoea
- Intestinal fistulae

- Ileostomy

- Vomiting due to High Intestinal Obstruction

- Decreased HCO3

- CO2 combing power

- Na+ and K+

Treatment

First treat the cause.

NS plus Hartman's Solution containing potassium and bicarbonate as lactate

Normal bicarbonate level HCO3 =24 (22–26 mEq/L)

Amount of bicarb required= 0.5 x weight in kg x (desired HCO3-Actual HCO3)

- 50% of this is replaced over 4 hours.

- Rest 50% is given over next 24 hours.

Precautions

i. Bolus doses should be avoided

ii. Never treat acidosis without treatment of aetiology

iii. Never treat acidosis without correction of associated Hypokalaemia as bicarbonate shifts Extracellular K+ to Intracellular K+- , further aggravates it

For Severe Acidosis–1.26% sodium bicarbonate–500 ml over 2 hours

ALKALOSIS–(DECREASED CHLORIDES)

Loss of Chlorides and decreased Na+ & k+

Increased Bicarbonate

Causes

1. Prolonged Vomiting
2. Prolonged Ryle's Tube Aspiration

Treatment

Normal Saline containing 3 gm of K+ as readymade solution.

Normal requirement of water, electrolytes, energy and protein.

Body Weight	Water (ml/kg/body wt.)	Sodium (mmol/kg/day	Potassium (mmol/kg/day)	Energy (Kcal/day)	Protein (g/day)
First 10 kgs	100	2–4	1.5–2.5	110	3.00
2nd 10 kgs	50	1–2	0.5–1.5	70	1.50
Subsequent weight in kgs	20	0.5–1	0.2–0.7	30	0.75

HYPOKALAEMIA– DECREASED POTASSIUM LEVEL IN BLOOD

Causes

1. In postoperative period increased loss of potassium in urine due to Na+ retention.

2. Prolonged I/V fluids in postoperative period

3. Excessive vomiting and diarrhoea

4. Increased dose of diuretics

Symptoms

Muscle cramps, Weakness.

T-wave change in ECG

Treatment

Kcl 10–20 mEq in 50 ml NS over one hour I/V x 4. This is fast-working treatment.

Maximum Replacement–20 mEq/hr I/V

20 mmol (1.5 gm) in normal saline is infused over the period of 4 hours.

Slow treatment consists of 1–2 gm potassium chloride/8 hourly for 24 hours, followed by 2 gms every 3–4 hrs until potassium level reaches normal.

Hypokalaemia and Hypomagnesaemia co-exist. So, treat hypomagnesia also.

There is little risk of hypokalaemia in the first 48 hours of the postoperative period.

There is always hypokalaemia if the patient is on prolonged I/V drip, for more than 48 hours.

Do not for wait for lab confirmation of deficiency for potassium replacement. Being mainly intracellular, it will not be accurately represented by the serum level.

Always administer potassium through normal saline because Dextrose solution may initially exacerbate hypokalaemia as a result of insulin mediated movement of potassium into cells.

HYPERKALAEMIA (RISE IN SERUM POTASSIUM LEVELS)

Causes

1. Excessive blood transfusion

2. Anaesthetic drugs

3. In renal failure patients

4. Excessive salt substitute

Symptoms

Weakness, Flaccid paralysis.

ECG–Peaked-T, Wide QRS and no P-Wave.

Treatment

- Inj. Calcium Gluconate-10 ml of 10%, I/V

- Injection-Bicarbonate (7.5 %)- 10 ml I/V

- Dextrose 50% (50 ml) given with 10–15 units of regular insulin I/V – it causes intracellular shift of potassium.

- Sodium Polystyrene Sulfonate–1 gm/kg as retention enema.

HYPERNATREMIA (INCREASED SODIUM IN SERUM)

Causes

In burn patients

In renal Failure

Symptoms

Confusion. Muscle tremors. Peripheral oedema.

Treatment

Hypovolemic Hypernatremia – Normal saline I/V to replace volume deficit, then Dextrose 5% to correct Hypernatremia.

Normovolemic Hypernatremia–Dextrose 5% is given/2 deficit first 24

hours and then the full amount within 48 hours.

HYPONATREMIA (DECREASED SODIUM IN SERUM)

Causes

Prolonged R.T Aspiration

Prolonged Vomiting and Diarrhoea

Treatment

When Serum Na^+ <130 mEq/lit

Neurological Signs (Na+ <120 mEq/lit)

→ treat promptly

What to give:

3% Nacl → 0.5 mEq Na+/ml

→ 2 – 3 ml/kg initial dose

→ use 3% Nacl to raise Na+ up to 125 mEq/lit

NaHco3 7.5% solution à 0.9 mEq Na+/ml

(if 3% Nacl not available)

		Dextrose gm/L	Na	K	Cl	Lactate	Ca	mOsm/L
Isotonic	NS		154		154			308
	RL		131	5	111	29	2	270
½ isotonic	½ NS		77		77			154
Electrolyte free solution	5% D	50						278
	10% D	100						556

		Dextrose gm/L	Na	K	Cl	Lactate	Ca	mOsm/L
Dextrose, electrolyte solution	**5% DNS**	50	154		154			585
	D 5 ½ NS	50	77		77			415
Paediatric Maint fluid	**Isolyte P**	50	25	20	22			368
	Isolyte M	50	40	35	38	Phosphate 15 meq/L Acetate 20		410
	Isolyte G	50	63	17	150	NH4CL 70		580

Solution	Concentration	Available from	Equivalents
Soda bicarb solution	7.5%	10 ml ampoule	1 ml = 1 mEq of HCO_3 + 1 mEq of Na
Potassium chloride	15% w/v	10 ml ampoule	1 ml = 2 mEq of K
Calcium gluconate	10% w/v	10 ml ampoule	1 ml = 9.3 mg of Cal.
Magnesium sulphate	50% and 25%	2 ml ampoule	If 25% Mg 4.15 mOsm/dL
Sodium chloride	3%	10 ml ampoule 50 ml bottle	1 ml = 0.5 mEq of Na

Take Home Message

Resuscitate with fluids early and aggressively.

It will neither overload nor will cause pulmonary oedema.

There are less likely hood for need of ICU.

Be guided by markers of tissue perfusion-

- **a. Urine output**
- **b. Lactate**
- **c. Corelate with central venous oxygen saturation**

How to make electrolyte water balance daily?

1. 1/4 tsp. salt.
2. 1/4 cup pomegranate juice.
3. 1/4 cup lemon juice.

4.1 1/2 cups unsweetened coconut water.

4.2 cups cold water.

Additional options: sweetener, powdered magnesium and/or calcium, depending on needs

REFERENCES

1. Viera AJ, Wouk N. Potassium Disorders: Hypokalaemia and Hyperkalaemia. Am Fam Physician. 2015 Sep 15;92(6):487-95.

2. Nagler EV, Vanmassenhove J, van der Veer SN, Nistor I, Van Biesen W, Webster AC et al. Diagnosis and treatment of hyponatremia: a systematic review of clinical practice guidelines and consensus statements. BMC Med. 2014 Dec 11;12:1. doi: 10.1186/s12916-014-0231-1. Review.

3. Walker MD. Fluid and Electrolyte Imbalances: Interpretation and Assessment. J Infus Nurs. 2016 Nov/Dec; 39(6):382-386.

Chapter 6

NUTRITION

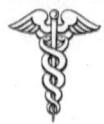

Pradeep Garg

Normal body nutrition is maintained by imbibing proteins carbohydrates, fats, vitamins, minerals and water. Malnutrition manifests in a majority (about 40–50%) of hospitalized patients. Nutritional support is essential for malnourished surgical patients. Sometimes, nutrition is required for healthy patients undergoing a major surgery.

The stress of surgery or trauma creates a hypermetabolic state, increasing protein and energy requirements. Macronutrients (fat, protein, and glycogen) from the labile reserves of fat tissue and skeletal muscle are redistributed to more metabolically active tissues such as the liver and visceral organs. This response can lead to the onset of protein-calorie malnutrition (defined as a negative balance of 100 g of nitrogen and 10,000 kcal) within a few days [1]. The rate of development of postoperative malnutrition in a given individual depends upon their pre-existing nutritional status, nature and complexity of the surgical procedure, and the degree of hypermetabolism.

Causes of malnutrition:

- Sepsis
- Multiple trauma and injuries
- Hypermetabolism and hyper catabolism
- Prolonged starvation
- Pre-existing malnourishment
- Severe haemorrhage and burns

Adverse effects of malnutrition: [2,3,4,5]:

- Increased frequency of decubitus ulcers
- Overgrowth of bacteria in the gastrointestinal tract
- Abnormal nutrient losses through stools
- Diminished wound healing
- Impaired immune function
- Increased chances of infection
- Retarded convalescence and increased hospital stay
- Higher mortality and morbidity rates

Role of good nutrition in critically ill patients:

- Decreased chances of infection
- Reduced incidence of morbidity and mortality

- Prevention and treatment of macro and micro nutrient deficiency

- Improved clinical outcome

Nutritional requirement for ICU patients per day:

- Energy–25 Kcal/kg/day

- Proteins/amino acids-1.2 to 1.5 g/kg/day

Total Parental Nutrition (TPN) is required in patients with major surgery and with multiple traumas.

CVP line is ideal for TPN infusion.

Blood sugar is checked every six hours.

Hyperglycaemia is controlled with insulin (sliding scale).

NORMAL REQUIREMENT

Total Volume - 2540 ml (1800 kcal)

1000 ml of amino acid plus 1000 ml of Dextrose 10% plus 500 ml of Fat emulsion (20%) plus 10 ml of 15% of Pot. Chloride plus 10 ml Na/K/Po4 additive.

MODERATELY INCREASED REQUIREMENT

Total Volume -3045 ml (2000 kcal)

1500 ml of Amino acid/Glucose plus 1000 ml of Dextrose 10% plus 500 ml of Fat emulsion (20%) plus 10 ml of Pot. Chloride (10 %) plus 15 ml of Na+/K+/Po4 additive

HIGHLY INCREASED REQUIREMENT

Total Volume - 2535 ml (2200 Kcal)

1000 ml Amino acid solution plus 500 ml of Dextrose 10 % plus Dextrose 50 % plus 500 ml of Fat emulsion (20 %) plus 15 ml of Na/K/Po4 additive.

ENTERAL NUTRITION

If there is peristalsis *it is advisable to use the gut for feeding.* There will be less chances of infection and the least post-operative complications. This is done by–

1. Ryle's Tube feeding, *if feeding is required for up to four weeks*

2. Gastrotomy or Percutaneous Endoscopic Gastrotomy (PEG), if feeding required more than four weeks

3. Feeding Jejunostomy

GASTRIC FEEDING

- Amount given is 25 ml/hour (Full strength fluids)

- If gastric residual is more than 150 ml then hold the feed for one hour and also give injectable/oral metoclopramide 6–8 hourly

- If gastric residual is less than 150 ml then increase the amount by 25 ml/hour increments every 8 hours

- Always elevate the head of bed for all patients who are receiving gastric tube feeding to avoid aspiration pneumonia due to regurgitation

- Flush the *Ryle's Tube* every four hours with water
- Methylene Blue may be added to feeding solution to identify aspiration in the lungs
- I/V fluids to be decreased accordingly

JEJUNAL FEEDING

- Same amount as gastric feeding
- No need for residual checking
- If nausea or distension occurs after feed then hold the feed
- Rate of feeding is increased by 10 ml/hour

Complications of Gastric Feeding

- Aspiration pneumonia
- Oesophigitis
- Sinusitis
- Loose motion

Take Home Message

1. The Role of Nutrition has great role in treatment of surgical patients.

2. A clear understanding of body's energy, fluids & electrolytes and micronutrients is essential to manage surgical patients.

3. Always try to use gut for enteral nutrition unless otherwise.

4. Parenteral nutrition only when enteral nutrition is contraindicated.

REFERENCES

1. Babineau TJ, Borlase BC, Blackburn GL. Applied Total Parental Nutrition in the Critically Ill. In: Intensive.

2. Mainous MR, Deitch EA. Nutrition and infection. Surg Clin North Am 1994; 74:659.

3. Care Medicine, Rippe JM, Irwin RS, Alpert JS, Fink MP (Eds), Little, Brown and Co, Boston 1991. p.1675.

4. Elwyn DH, Bryan-Brown CW, Shoemaker WC. Nutritional aspects of body water dislocations in postoperative and depleted patients. Ann Surg 1975; 182:76.

5. Kinney JM, Weissman C. Forms of malnutrition in stressed and unstressed patients. Clin Chest Med 1986; 7:19.

Chapter 7

BLOOD TRANSFUSION AND BLOOD PRODUCTS

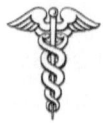

Ranabir Pal

"Despite all the technological marvels that humanity is experiencing, a reliable and safe blood supply, is still out of reach for untold millions of people around the world."

- GH Brundtland, Director General, WHO

DEFINITION OF BLOOD TRANSFUSION

A procedure in which whole blood or parts of blood are transfused into a patient's bloodstream through a vein. The blood may be donated by another person or it may have been taken from the patient and stored until needed (auto-transfusion).

Ethical transfer of blood and blood products from donor to recipient is typically done to save lives by replacing the component of blood reduced by injury, pathophysiological reasons or during surgical interventions, to bring back homeostasis. The safest blood product is that which is taken from same person and later transfused, which is only possible in planned operative manoeuvres as per the systems approach of clinical practice guidelines. We need safe blood transfusion services from interprofessional, ethically coordinated team approach, starting from need assessment through correct documentation to the site of blood collection from non-remunerated altruistic donors and transfusion to the correct recipient, while taking care of intra and post transfusion hazards viz. fever, chills, dyspnoea, itching, or general discomfort.

INDICATION OF TRANSFUSION

a. Acute blood loss (RBCs containing components are given)

b. Critical haemostatic failure (Platelets, plasma or whole blood is given)

AIM OF TRANSFUSION THERAPY

a. To maintain circulatory volume

b. Adequate oxygen delivery to tissues

RECIPIENTS OF BLOOD TRANSFUSION

There are several surgical reasons for blood transfusions, ranging from cardiothoracic surgery, injuries, etc. and medical reasons, from severe acute or chronic infections, liver and kidney diseases, cancer, congenital and acquired causes, to affect haematogenesises.

Pre-Operative Autologous Transfusion: The blood is drawn from the patient before surgery and stored till the same person needs it during or after non-emergency (elective) surgery. Advantage: Eliminate the need of other's help and any mismatch during transfusion. Disadvantage: Exclusively used with planned surgery that may incur postponement; not possible in emergency medical conditions.

Intra-Operative Autologous Transfusion: Blood is recycled during surgery by filtering the lost amount during the operation and intraoperatively putting it back into the patient's body. Advantage: Large amounts of blood can be transfused in both emergency and elective surgeries with the above-mentioned advantages; suitable in the presence of cancer or infections.

Post-Operative Autologous Transfusion: The amount of blood lost during surgery is collected and transfused to same patient after doing processing of collected bloodafter emergency and elective surgeries. Advantage: Comparable to intra-operative autologous transfusion.

Haemodilution: In the immediate preoperative period, the blood is collected and surgery done with intravenous fluids; postoperatively the same blood is transfused after processing. Advantage: In this process during elective surgeries, the person loses diluted blood, but post-operatively it is replaced by pure autologous blood with minimum hassles.

Apheresis: The process of self-donation of plasma and platelets with limited danger. Advantage: This method is comparable to intra-operative autologous transfusion. Disadvantage: Restricted quantity of blood is drawn anticipating severe blood loss post-operatively in elective surgeries, which limits universal application.

DONORS FOR BLOOD TRANSFUSION

Donated blood is rigorously tested for safe transfusion, though the battery of screening methods cannot nullify all hazards. Two types of donations need to be mentioned:

NON-REMUNERATED DONORS: Blood banks collect blood from healthy volunteer altruistic donors. There is a higher probability of availability tempered with transfusion hazards.

DESIGNATED DONORS: Blood is collected from a selected donor from the community, instead of unknown donors. Comparable risks include the possibility of allergic reaction and procedural delay.

BLOOD GROUP

Almost all corpuscles, including red blood cells, have multiple surface molecules that have properties of immunological cellular interactions. These multiple reacting sites on each cell, made from groups of related molecules, are ultimately expressed as the blood group of the individual, which is genetically inherited viz. Rh or the ABO systems. Thus the red blood cell types of the donor and the recipient must match, in order to avoid life-threatening post-transfusion reactions.

Four major blood types viz. A (with A-antigen and anti-B-antibody), B (with B-antigen and anti-A-antibody), AB (with both A and B antigen and no comparable antibody), or O (with no A and B antigen with both anti-A and anti-B-antibodies); Rh-typing makes them Rh-positive, or -negative. For example, B group blood is either Type B Rh-positive or Type B Rh-negative. Though a person with Type O blood has the classic nomenclature of universal donors, yet it's preferable to use the same blood group in non-emergency situations. On the contrary, individuals with Type AB blood are called universal recipients though same group is usually preferred unless in emergency situations. Rh-typing is more rigorously considered in transfusion services, except in life-threatening situations.

BLOOD COMPONENTS

Whole blood transfusion is out of practice now-a-days. Instead, blood is transfused usually as components depending on the specific medical and surgical needs of the recipient.

RED BLOOD CELLS: The most commonly transfused components are packed red cells to improve tissue oxygen supply in cases of trauma or surgical loss of blood or severe anaemia or toxaemia.

PLATELETS AND CLOTTING FACTORS: In bleeding diathesis of unknown or known aetiologies including internal exsanguination, inherited bleeding disorder or hemoglobinopathies.

PLASMA: Fresh frozen plasma is commonly used as a volume expander due to acute injury from burn, trauma, etc.

BLOOD TRANSFUSION SERVICES

Before Transfusion

National Blood Policy (2002) issued by the Government of India has provided guidelines for the quality and quantity of safe transfusion of blood components and products collected from non-remunerated volunteer blood donors. Healthcare personnel should sincerely follow these guidelines in letter and spirit, which regulate the process of blood transfusion. From assessing eligibility, to collection, to blood grouping and cross-matching – everything should be done to transfuse blood which minimizes medical problems during and after transfusion. These guidelines include donor and recipient criteria, necessary processing of donated blood, storage and precautions in the blood transfusion services.

During Transfusion

Healthcare delivery systems must ensure that clinical practice guidelines are followed and that trained healthcare personnel verify details of the recipients and blood, for the safety of the recipients. These include prevention of wrong cross-matching, tests for HIV, Hepatitis B and C, infections, etc., followed by proper volume and proper rate with clear orders for monitoring the pulse, BP, temperature, respiratory rate, and other anticipatory signs of mismatched blood transfusion.

After Transfusion

After transfusion, all vital signs are checked for transfusion related reactions by a dedicated, trained, healthcare team for appropriate signs and symptoms.

TRANSFUSION RELATED MEDICAL ISSUES

Allergic Reactions: Allergic reactions may occur even when the transfusion process follows all aspects rigidly. The symptoms could be mild (itching, chills, flushing) to severe (shock), that should be urgently addressed to optimise the safety of the recipient.

Communicable Diseases: The transfusion services routinely screened donated blood for microbial contaminations viz. HIV, Hepatitis B and C, Malaria and syphilis before processing and storage. After suitable screening, the blood should be transfused and the healthcare team should be mindful regarding transfusion related infections.

Fever: Chills and fever, during or within a day of blood transfusion occur as the body's normal response to leukocytes which blood banks may remove, to reduce this post- transfusion reaction.

Iron Overload: From repeated blood transfusions, iron molecules may build up in thalassemia, that may damage the liver, heart, and other parts (hemochromatosis), which need chelation therapy.

Lung Injury: Dyspnoea, arising from the uncertain aetiology of the damage to lung cells, usually occurs within six hours of transfusion, which may be fatal for up to one in four cases. Risk factors for lung injury are - being very ill pre-transfusion, pregnant, etc.

Acute immune haemolytic reaction: Haemolytic reaction is serious though rare in a mismatched transfusion - with symptoms that include chill, fever, nausea, vomiting, chest pain, dark urine - for which we need to immediately discontinue transfusion at the first sign.

Delayed haemolytic reaction: This chronic problem may be unnoticed until anaemia sets in, which is commonly noted in patients with previous as well as repeated transfusions.

Graft-Versus-Host disease: This condition is usually fatal, triggered by leukocytes, in immune-compromised patients, within one month of transfusion, presenting features of fever, rash, diarrhoea.

Complication	Signs/Symptoms	Treatment	Extraneous
Febrile Transfusion Reaction	1 degree rise in temp. May have chills, malaise	Supportive - acetaminophen	Most Common
Hemolytic Transfusion Reaction	Fever, chills, pain at the site of reaction, nausea/ vomiting, shock, dark urine	STOP the transfusion Lots of IV fluids +/- diuretcs	Worst reaction. Often a clerical issue - ABO incompatibility
Allergic Reaction	Urticaria, pruritis, hives. Anaphylaxis is rare	Symptomatic - antihistamines. Do NOT need to stop transfusion	Note: they are not actually allergic to blood but secondary to antibodies in the blood
TRALI (Transfusion Related Acute Lung Injury)	dyspnea, hypoxemia, bilateral chest infiltrates (think ARDS)	STOP the transfusion - airway control, supportive care	Most common cause of death associated with transfusions but..better prognosis than most ARDS
TACO (Transfusion Associated Circulatory Overload)	dyspnea, edema	Give blood slowly (over 3-4 hours) Diuretics with transfusion	Often occurs in the elderly and chronically anemic

ESSENTIAL ISSUES

Notes

a. If haemoglobin is less than 7 gm/dl then it means that the patient cannot tolerate acute blood loss and there is high mortality during surgery. Yet, replacing all blood loss with transfusion is a wasteful practice that exposes the recipient to unnecessary risk of massive transfusion.

b. Up to 500 ml of blood can be lost rapidly, without ill effects on the body. 1–2 litres of fluid loss does not cause hypotension.

c. Children/Elderly/Cardiac/Pulmonary patients have less resistance to blood loss and are also more prone to suffer problems arising from over transfusion.

d. H/O Aspirin intake or anticoagulant is very important as Aspirin causes irreversible platelets dysfunction. Doing PTI and platelets count is essential. Major surgery should be delayed for about one week if the patient is on Aspirin. If emergency surgery is to be done on such a patient, then give them an infusion of platelets.

e. Always look for coagulopathy in the post-operative period as, after massive blood loss and fluid replacement, an acquired coagulopathy can arise due to delusional thrombocytopenia and dilution of soluble clotting factors. Platelets transfusion helps in treating patients with coagulopathy.

f. Plasma (1 litre in adults) helps to replace clotting factors

PLATELETS TRANSFUSION

Volume approximately 175 ml per 10 units; each unit should raise platelets ten thousands; Cross match unnecessary, yet ABO and Rh compatibility recommended.

CLOTTING FACTOR TRANSFUSION

Patients with specific clotting factor deficiency require that specific factor replacement. Usually this means 'Fresh Frozen Plasma'. If the patient is on Warfarin and requires urgent surgery then administer Clotting Factor concentrate (II, IX, X, XI factors).

FRESH FROZEN PLASMA

Contains all coagulation factors including 200 units of factor 8 per unit; Indicated for bleeding due to elevated PT/PTI; No cross-matching but ABO compatibility must.; each unit contains 150–200 ml volume and usually 4–6 units required at a time.

CRYOPRECIPITATE

Indicated in Haemophilia A, low fibrinogen, post-cardiopulmonary bypass to correct coagulopathy. Each unit contains factor VIII, XIII, von Willebrand's factor , fibrinogen and fibronectin; 8–10 units are required at a time; No cross matching required.

PACKED RED BLOOD CELLS

Indicated for haemorrhage; 300–350 ml per unit; Deficient in platelets and clotting factors.

WHOLE BLOOD

450 ml per unit; Typing and cross matching required; Deficient in platelets and factor V, VII, XI.

Take Home Message

To sum up, ultimately a scientifically sound, interprofessional team approach should be instituted to optimize blood transfusion services. We need standard office procedures at each step - from motivating voluntary donations though collection, component separation, storage and transfusion practices, to the right recipient at right time with right quality at right quantity following right process.

REFERENCES

1. These were the Words of Dr. Brundtland GH, Director-General of the World Health Organization, at the launch of World Health Day 2000 dedicated to Blood Safety. [online] Available from: http://hinfo.humaninfo.ro/gsdl/health techdocs/documents/s15376e/s15376e. pdf. [Last accessed Aug., 2019]

2. Medicine Net Blood Transfusion Procedure, Reactions, Risks, Side Effects, Complications. Medical Author: Jerry R. Balentine, DO, FACEP Medical Editor: Jay W. Marks, M.

Chapter 8

PREOPERATIVE ASSESSMENT AND PREPARATION FOR ANAESTHESIA AND SURGERY

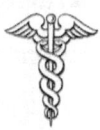

Jagdish Dureja

Preoperative medical assessment is done by the anaesthetist to minimize the patient's surgical and anaesthetic perioperative morbidity or mortality.

STEPS OF PREOPERATIVE VISIT

* 1. Doctor Patient Relationship
* 2. Patient Data
* 3. Problems Identification
* 4. Patient consent
* 5. Preopeartive Preparation
* 6. Plan of anesthetic Techniques

Preoperative evaluation and preparation is done as follows: [1,2]

1. Name of surgical procedure.

2. Checking of all relevant investigations desired for that surgical procedure and assessment of the patient's health.

3. Determination of perioperative risks.

4. Preoperative correction of the patient's medical condition.

5. Total explanation to the patient about surgery, anaesthesia, intraoperative care and postoperative care.

Patient Pre-anaesthesia Check Up

1. Proper History

2. Physical Examination

3. Lab Workup: Special Tests

Lab tests should be ordered based on the information obtained from the history and physical exam, the age of the patient and the type of surgery. [3, 4, 5, 6]

4. Drug History

5. Perioperative Risk Assessment:

Assessment for Abdominal Surgery (Non traumatic cases):-

The American Society of Anaesthesiology (*ASA*) *grading system* is the gold standard to assess a patient's physical state and should be applied to all patients who come for surgery. [7,8] Emergency surgery increases risks dramatically, especially in patients in ASA class 4 and 5.

(ASA) scale is used to measure a patient's well-being.

ASA-1--Healthy patient (no other disease) 0 % mortality.

ASA-2--One system disease well controlled and does not affect daily activity (predict minimal mortality).

ASA-3--Multisystem disease, but well controlled, limits activity (predict some increased mortality).

ASA 4–Severe incapacitating disease with poor control, constant threat to life (greatly increased mortality predicted).

ASA5–Moribund patient not expected to survive 24 hours with or without surgery.

ASA6–Brain dead organ donor.

Subclass E–indicates emergent procedure. Emergency surgeries increase mortality by 50%.

IN TRAUMA PATIENTS UNDERGOING LAPAROTOMY

Preoperative assessment is as follows:

a. Respiratory rate-

10–24/Minutes----4 points

25–35/Minutes----3

>35/Minutes------2

<10/Minutes-------1

       0/Minute--------0

  b. Respiratory efforts-

      Normal----1 point

      Shallow or reactive–0

  c. Blood Pressure-

      90–100 mm Hg-----4 points

      70–90 mm Hg--------3

      50–69 mm Hg--------2

      < 50 mm Hg---------1

      Not recordable--------0

  d. Capillary Refill-

      Normal-----2 points

      Delayed------1

GLASGOW COMA SCALE

Eye Opening:

Spontaneous—4

To voice---------3

To pain----------2

None----------1

Verbal Response:

Oriented----------5

Confused---------4

Inappropriate words–3

Incomprehensive words-----2

None-------1

Motor Response:

Obey command—6

Purposeful movement–5

Withdrawal--------4

Flexion-------------3

Extension-----------2

None-------------1

GCS Code:

14–15------------5

11–13------------4

8–10-------------3

5–7---------------2

So total trauma score is A+B+C+D+E. Higher the score the better the prognosis.

It is most important to decrease the interval between the time of injury and definite care and surgical procedure. So the first hour is called the Golden Hour.

1. So, in an emergency, immediate surgical consultation and operation within the first hour, is lifesaving - especially in cases of intra peritoneal hemorrhage due to liver and spleen injury, rupture of aortic aneurism, etc.

2. Urgent surgery means within 4 to 6 hours – for instance, all gut perforations requiring surgery and cases of intestinal obstruction.

Other factors to be considered in preoperative period are:

Age–More than 40 years– morbidity increases

CVS system

Coronary artery disease, CHF, Arrhythmias, Hypertension. All these increase morbidity and mortality.

Cardiac risk following MI

0–3 months--------up to 10 %

4–6 months---------up to 3 %

>6 months----------up to 1%

History of bleeding disorders is very important.

RESPIRATORY SYSTEM – [9]

Postoperative pulmonary complications (PPCs) like pneumonia, atelectasis, bronchitis, bronchospasm, occur in approximately 20–30% of patients undergoing major, non-thoracic surgery. So, an assessment of the respiratory system is equally essential.

Pulmonary Risk Factors:

- Age>65

- Obesity - increases the morbidity

- Tobacco using history– > than 15 years and one pack/day increases the morbidity multifold

- Prolonged hospitalization

- *Procedure-related risk factors:* primarily based on how close the surgery is to the diaphragm (i.e. upper abdominal and thoracic surgery are procedures with the highest risk)

- *Length of surgery* (> 3 hours) and general anaesthesia (vs. epidural or spinal)

- Emergency surgery

- Asthma and COPD increase morbidity

- Presence of obstructive sleep apnoea

- Poor exercise tolerance or poor general health status

RENAL SYSTEM

- Blood Urea > than 50 mgs%

- Serum Creatinine > than 3 mgs%

Increases morbidity

HEPATIC SYSTEM

- Active hepatitis and cirrhosis of liver increases morbidity

ENDOCRINE SYSTEM

- Diabetes Mellitus

- Thyroid Disease

- Steroid Therapy

All the above increase morbidity and mortality.

So, pre-operatively gathering a detailed history about all the above comorbidity is essential.

- Proper physical examination from head to toe, including genitalia.

- Per rectal and per vaginal examination is mandatory.

INVESTIGATIONS

- Routine Haemograms (Hb should be >than 10 gms)

- Total Blood Counts

- Blood Sugar - Fasting and postprandial

- Blood Urea and Sr. Creatinine

- LFT

- Serum Electrolytes

- Complete Urine

- Blood Grouping

- PTI, INR

- ECG - if the age is > than 40 years

- X-Ray Chest

- Viral markers

  Patient should be afebrile.

  Empty stomach more than 6 hours.

  Hydration of the patient should be normal.

Neutralize the gastric acid with antacids.

Avoid blood transfusion in chronically anaemic patients.

Correction of electrolytes and metabolic acidosis.

CONTROL OF DIABETES MELLITUS

Morbidity and mortality rates are higher in diabetic than in non-diabetic patients in the perioperative phase. Diabetics have a higher incidence of death after MI, than non-diabetics. Myocardial ischemia or infarction may be clinically "silent" if the diabetic has autonomic neuropathy. Therefore, a high index of suspicion for myocardial ischemia or infarction should be maintained throughout the perioperative period if unexplained hypotension, dysrhythmias, hypoxemia or ECG changes develop. [10,11] The diabetic patient undergoing elective surgery should be carefully evaluated preoperatively for symptoms and signs of peripheral vascular, cerebrovascular and coronary disease.

PER OPERATIVE MANAGEMENT OF ANTICOAGULANT

There is a high risk of hemorrhage and an increasing risk of thromboembolism (venous, arterial) after discontinuing oral anticoagulation therapy, and there is no consensus as to how perioperative anticoagulation should be managed. [12,13,14,15]

1. Most patients can undergo dental extractions, arthrocentesis, biopsies, ophthalmic operations

and diagnostic endoscopy without alteration of their anticoagulant regimen. For other invasive and surgical procedures, oral anticoagulation needs to be withheld and the decision whether to pursue an aggressive strategy of perioperative administration of intravenous (IV) heparin or subcutaneous (SC) low-molecular-weight heparin (LMWH), vary from patient to patient.

2. Invasive surgery is generally safe (from major haemorrhagic complications) when the INR ~1.5. Approximately four days is needed for the INR to reach 1.5 once the oral anticoagulant is stopped preoperatively.

3. It takes approximately three days for the INR to reach 2.0 once the oral anticoagulant is restarted postoperatively.

4. If the oral anticoagulant is withheld four days pre-op and started immediately post-op, the patient is, in the meantime, without anticoagulation for two days (24 hours preop and 24 hours post-op).

Management recommendations: [16,17]

1. If INR pre-op is 2–3, stop oral anticoagulant four days prior to surgery (or longer if INR > 3.0).

2. Measure INR one day prior to surgery: if it is ≥ 1.7, give 1 mg vitamin K SC.

3. If on the day of surgery the INR is 1.3–1.7, administer 1 unit of fresh frozen plasma and administer 2 units if the INR is 1.7–2.0.

4. The following approaches can be used: administer full-dose anticoagulation with IV

unfractionated heparin (UFH); administer full-dose anticoagulation with LMWH; or administer prophylactic doses of UFH or LMWH.

Patients receiving fibrinolytic/thrombolytic medications are at a risk of serious haemorrhagic events:

1. Following a lumbar puncture, spinal or epidural anaesthesia, or epidural steroid injection, thrombolytic drugs should be avoided for at least ten days.

2. No clear data is available to outline the length of time a neuraxial puncture should be avoided after discontinuation of these drugs.

Patient on Unfractionated Heparin in preoperative period (UFH)

UFH is monitored with the help of activated partial thromboplastin time (aPTT). Normal values of the aPTT range from 24 to 35 s.

Patient Receiving Low Molecular Weight Heparin (LMWH)

LMWH is used as prophylaxis of postsurgical deep vein thrombosis (DVT). Dose of enoxaparin is 30 mg SC every 12 hours, with the initial dose administered 12–24 hours postoperatively.

Nonsteroidal Anti-Inflammatory Drugs (NSAIDs), antiplatelet medications and spinal axis anaesthesia:

NSAIDS alter platelet function and may increase the risk of spinal/epidural hematoma formation if spinal axis anesthesia is utilized without following proper precautions.

Patients receiving aspirin or NSAID:

1. The use of COX-1 or COX-2 NSAIDs alone does not create a level of risk that will interfere with the performance of neuraxial blocks.

2. According to European Societies, there is a risk of hematoma formation when these agents are used in the perioperative period and they recommend that at least a 3-day interval without aspirin, or aspirin containing medication, before neuraxial blocks are performed or epidural catheters are removed. In addition, they also recommend a 1–2 day drug-free interval for all other COX-1 NSAIDs.

Patients receiving antiplatelet drugs:

ASRA guidelines are as follows:-

1. Ticlopidine (Ticlid) should be discontinued 14 days prior to surgery.

2. It is recommended that clopidogrel (Plavix) be stopped 7 days prior to surgery.

Patients receiving platelet Glycoprotein IIb/IIIa Antagonists:

ASRA guidelines are as follows:-

1. Abciximab should be discontinued 48 hours prior to surgery.

2. It is recommended that Eptifibatide and Tirofiban be stopped 8 hours prior to surgery.

If patient is on Aspirin, then, ideally stop the drug 7–8 days prior to surgery. Minimum gap required is 72 hours.

Pre-Operative Antibiotics–Broad spectrum like 3rd/4th generation Cephalosporins

- Vancomycin 1 gm I/V in penicillin allergic patients.

- Amino glycosides if renal functions are normal.

- Metrogyl for abdominal and pelvic surgery.

Bowel Preparation – Ideally 6 hours of fasting. Sips of plain water can be given up to two hours before surgery.

An empty colon is essential before colonic surgery as the colon is full of faeces (bacteria). But right hemicolectomy can be done on an unprepared bowel. In case of left side colonic surgery, bowel preparation is done 36 hours before definite surgery by an oral preparation of Ethylene glycol or Sodium Picosulphate.

In case of intestinal obstruction intraoperative on-table lavage is performed.

These days no preoperative antibiotics like Neomycin and Erythromycin are given as they carry the risk of intestinal super infection with yeast and resistant bacteria.

Take Home Message

Preanesthesia examination is as important as a well done surgery

REFERENCES

1. Roizen MF, Foss JF, Fischer SP. Preoperative evaluation. In: Miller RD, editor. Anaesthesia.

5th Edition. Philadelphia: Churchill-Livingstone; 2000. pp. 824–883.

2. Kitts JB. The preoperative assessment; who is responsible? Can J Anesth. 1997; 44:1232, 1236. [PubMed]

3. American Society of Anaesthesiologists Task Force on Preanesthesia Evaluation Practice Advisory for Preanesthesia Evaluation. Anaesthesiology. 2002; 96:485–496. [PubMed]

4. Roizen MF. Preoperative laboratory testing: What is needed? 54th ASA Annual Refresher Course Lectures. 2003:146.

5. Halaszynski TM, Juda R, Silverman DG. Optimizing postoperative outcomes with efficient preoperative assessment and management. Crit Care Med. 2004;32:S80. [PubMed]

6. Rabkin SW, Horne JM. Preoperative Electrocardiography: effect of new abnormalities on clinical decisions. Can Med Asso J. 1983; 128:146. [PMC free article] [PubMed]

7. Fleisher LA. Risk of anaesthesia. In: Miller RD, editor. Anaesthesia. 5th Edition. Philadelphia: Churchill-Livingstone; 2000. pp. 795–823.

8. Cohen MM, Duncan PG, Tate RB. Does anaesthesia contribute to operative mortality? JAMA.1988;260:2859. [PubMed]

9. Smetana GW. Current concepts: preoperative pulmonary evaluation. N.Engl.J. Med. 1999;340:937–944. [PubMed]

10. Coursin DB. Perioperative management of the diabetic patient. 55th ASA Annual Refresher Course Lectures. 2004:210.

11. Juul AB, Wetterslev J, Kofoed-Enevoldsen A, et al. The Diabetic Postoperative Mortality and Morbidity (DIPOM) trial: Rationale and design of a multicentre, randomized, placebo-controlled, clinical trial of metoprolol for patients with diabetes mellitus who are undergoing major noncardiac surgery. American Heart Journal. 2004; 147:677–683. [PubMed]

12. Kearon C, Hirsh J. Perioperative Management of Patients Receiving Oral Anticoagulants. Arch Intern Med. 2003; 163:2532–2533. [PubMed]

13. Eckman MH. "Bridging On the River Kwai": The Perioperative Management of Anticoagulation Therapy. Med Decis Making. 2005; 25:370–373. [PubMed]

14. Dunn AS, Wisnivesky J. Perioperative Management of Patients on Oral Anticoagulants: A Decision Analysis. Med Decis Making. 2005; 25:387–397. [PubMed]

15. Kovacs MJ, Kearon C, Rodger M, et al. Single-arm study of bridging therapy with low-molecular-weight heparin for patients at risk of arterial embolism who require temporary interruption of warfarin. Circulation.2004;110:1658–1663. [PubMed]

16. Broadman LM. Anticoagulation and regional anaesthesia. 55th ASA Annual Refresher Course Lectures.2004:248.

17. Horlocker TT, Wedel DJ, Benzon H, et al. Regional anaesthesia in the anticoagulated patient: Defining the risks (The Second ASRA Consensus Conference on Neuraxial Anaesthesia and Anticoagulation) Reg Anes and Pain Med. 2003;28:172–197. [PubMed]

Chapter 9

POST-OPERATIVE MANAGEMENT

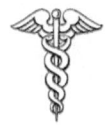

Nivesh Agarwal

Postoperative care starts at the end of the operation and carries on in the postoperative period. Hypotension, airway protection, pain control, urinary retention, <u>deep venous thrombosis</u> (DVT), mental status, constipation and wound healing are the major worries in the postoperative period. Blood glucose levels should be monitored closely every 1–4 hours for diabetes patients until the patients start eating.

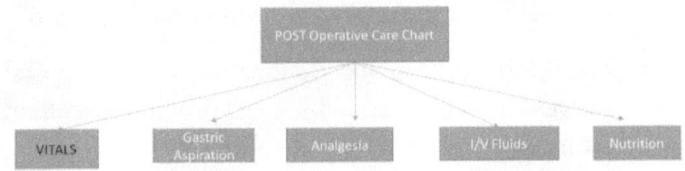

Postoperative care is very important for full recovery of patient after a successful surgical procedure and the surgeon has to be alert for:

- Position of patient in bed

- Proper bedding condition to avoid bed sores

- Care of wound/stomas/fistulae

- Care of catheter/Ryle's tube/drains

- Care of central venous line

- Physiotherapy and compressible stockings to avoid deep vein thrombosis

Pain relief in postoperative period is very important as chest movements are good in a pain-free patient and thus there are less chances of chest infection/nausea/hypotensive episodes and also post-operative ileus.

Postoperative pain relief:

- In day care patients – Oral NSAID with paracetamol and codeine sulphate, are good analgesics. Drugs can be started before surgery.

- Local infiltration of anaesthetic drugs (bupivacaine) is done in wounds to provide good pain relief for 4–6 hours in postoperative period.

- Local infiltration of Xylocaine in intercostal nerves in fractured ribs will provide excellent pain relief.

- Intramuscular injections of opiates, given every 4–6 hours as bolus injections, provide pain relief for 24–48 hours. But they produce widely fluctuating levels of pain relief, so, Patient Controlled Analgesia (PCA) is a better option.

- Intravenous opiate is given as 2.5 mgs of Morphine. It gives the fastest pain relief and can be repeated at 5 to 10 minute intervals, with maximum dose of up to 10 mgs.

Patient Controlled Analgesia (PCA)

In this, the dose is controlled by the patient. Here, the opiate is given intravenously. The patient can give himself the drug as a bolus dose (1 mg) by pressing the button. But the risk of overdose has to be kept in mind. The delivery system has got various safety lockout features, in-built, to avoid rapid delivery of repeated bolus doses.

Hazards:

- Overdosing
- Accidental pressing by child visitors

Epidural Analgesia:

- very good method
- complete pain-free postoperative period in abdominal and thoracic surgery
- Maximum period 46–72 hours

Drawbacks:

- Overdose leading to hypertension
- Blockade of epidural catheter result in severe pain, which is sometimes difficult to control

- Infection in epidural space

- A hematoma at the insertion site can result in irreversible cord damage

Contraindications:

- in patients with clotting abnormalities

- in patients on heparin therapy

Intravenous Fluids Replacement:

Patients who have undergone abdominal surgery will require I/V fluids in the post-operative period.

First post-operative day:

In young adults– Total 2–3 litres is given (1 litre of Saline and 2 litres of 5% Dextrose)

In elderly patients– total 2 litres (500 ml of Saline and 1.5 litres of Dextrose)

These solutions are also available with potassium chloride (40 mmol/litre)

Give more fluid in summer to compensate for increased sweating

Input/output Chart must be maintained

Daily balance should be about 1000 cc

Second post-operative day:

Same as above. Replace Isolyte-G for gastric aspiration and Isolyte-M for maintenance.

B-Complex (vitamins) must be added from the second day of postoperative care

Maintenance Regime:

80 kgs - young man —

2 litres Dextrose + 1 litre Saline +(81 mmol of potassium + 1.5 to 2 mmol/kg of sodium)

40 kgs - old woman—

1.5 litres Dextrose + 500 ml Saline + (54 mmol of potassium + 1.5 to 2 mmol of sodium)

A fall in serum potassium is a late indicator of depletion of total body potassium which is mainly intracellular. Potassium should be replaced even if the serum potassium is within the normal range.

NUTRITION IN POSTOPERATIVE PERIOD

Nutritional failure is also one of the contributory factors for morbidity and mortality in the postoperative period. It has got special relevance in G.I. surgery. Solution of amino acids, glucose and emulsions of lipids form the basis of IV feeding. All the constituents are mixed in a single bag and to this are added electrolytes, vitamins and trace elements.

Normal requirements-(Energy-1800 Kcal)

(Volume–2540 ml) –1000 ml of Amino acids and Glucose + 1000 ml of 10 % Dextrose + 500 ml of 20 % Fat emulsion +10 ml of 15 % potassium chloride + 10 ml of Na/K+/PO4 additive.

Moderately increased requirement — (Energy–2000 Kcal)

(Volume–3045 ml)—1500 ml Amino acids/glucose +1000 ml of 10% Dextrose +500 ml of 20% Fat emulsion

+ 10 ml of 10% potassium chloride + 15 ml of Na+/K+/ PO4 additive.

Greatly increased requirement:

(Volume–2500 ml)-----1000 ml of Amino acids + 500 ml of 10% Dextrose + 500 ml of 50% Dextrose + 500 ml of 20% Fat emulsion + 15 ml of Na+/K+/PO4 additive.

Care of Patients receiving IV nutrition:

- Care of central venous line
- Care of patient's metabolic state
- C.V. line - dressing is changed every seven days.
- Skin around the catheter is cleaned with antiseptic lotion.
- Look for infection. Treat if present.
- Avoid mechanical damage of catheter by proper, gentle handling.
- Infusion equipment should function properly.

CARE OF PATIENT'S METABOLIC STATE

—Regular weighing

----S/S of fluid depletion/overload

Daily Check–serum electrolyte, urea, creatinine, glucose level

Twice a week—serum albumin, protein, calcium, magnesium, phosphate. Liver function tests

Complications

- Glucose disturbance, Lipid disturbances, Nitrogen disturbances

- Ventilator problems – excessive amount of glucose can cause increased production of carbon dioxide resulting in failure of ventilator

GASTRIC ASPIRATION

Advantages

Keeping the stomach empty is very important in peri-operative period to avoid chances of aspiration and thus, lung infection. In G.I. Surgeries, Ryle's tube aspiration is necessary to treat paralytic ileus. It also helps in relieving gaseous distension.

Disadvantages

- The tube can provoke vomiting and inhalation

- Feeling of foreign body in nasopharynx and pharynx

- Inhibit coughing and thus can cause stasis of lung's excretions

- Lately, oesophageal stricture

- Due to its narrow calibre, the Ryle's tube may fail to remove semisolid material, so there's no guarantee that the patient will not vomit

Technique of inserting Ryle's tube – Standard Nasogastric tube:

The tube should have 3 mm internal bore for adult patients. A little cotton soaked in 4% Lignocaine should be applied to mucosa just within the external nostril. Well lubricate the tube with Xylocaine jelly and pass it horizontally backwards with one hand while supporting the head with the other. When the tube goes into the nasopharynx, ask the patient to swallow and give him sips of water. Check the position by putting 20 cc air and auscultate over stomach. Fix the tube to the nose with an adhesive plaster.

The Nasogastric tube should be removed as early as possible:

- if the aspirate is less than 300–400 per day
- When the aspirate is clear and odourless
- When bowel sounds are present
- Patient has passed flatus

Block the tube. Give 50 ml of water hourly and at the end of 3–4 hours. If aspirated volume is less than half, then remove the Ryle's tube.

HICCOUGHS

- A sign of gastric dilation
- A sign of irritation of the diaphragm as in sub diaphragmatic sepsis
- In cases of uraemia

Treatment—Ryle's tube aspiration

- I/V Injection Chlorpromazine and Pethidine 25 mg each in divided doses

- Carbo dioxide inhalation may be tried
- Usually self-limiting

COMPLICATIONS IN POST-OPERATIVE PERIOD

Respiratory System

A. Atelectasis - This is most likely cause of post-operative fever in the first 48–72 hours. The alveoli collapse due to inadequate lung expansion as a result of post-operative pain and this results in decreased movement of the diaphragm. Due to pain, coughing is suppressed which impairs clearing of lung secretions, thus causing atelectasis.

S/S-Fever, Tachycardia, Tachypnoea and decreased sounds on bases of lungs.

Management:

   a. Adequate analgesia

   b. Early ambulation in post-operative period

   c. Deep breathing

   d. Chest percussion and postural drainage

   e. Prophylactic antibiotics like Injection Amoxicillin 500 mgs for 4 weeks to avoid secondary infection with Haemophilus influenzae

B Adult respiratory distress syndrome (ARDS) – Diffuse lung injury which occurs 24–72 hrs. in post-operative period.

Due to high intra-abdominal pressure, narcotics overdose, atelectasis, pneumonia, pulmonary oedema, hypovolemia, there is inadequate tissue oxygenation (decreased pulmonary gas exchange)

S/S–respiratory rate >25 or <10, confusion, agitation, cyanosis as pO_2 <60 and pCO_2 >50

Management—Mechanical Ventilation

C Pneumonia—Due to pain, there is stagnation of secretion in lower respiratory tract and normal inhabitants (commensals) of upper tract reign supreme and cause pneumonia. Treatment is physiotherapy, antibiotics, tracheal toilet and bronchoscopy.

D Pulmonary Embolism–This is due to a blood clot lodging in the pulmonary artery. Blood clots usually arise from deep veins thrombosis on calf veins, thigh veins, iliac or pelvic veins.

Predisposing factors –* immobility * pelvic surgery

S/S–Sudden chest pain and dyspnoea

Tachypnoea and Hypotension

Definite diagnosis is by pulmonary angiography.

Management–1) Heparin anticoagulant, 2) Cardio-respiratory support in I C U 3) Embolectomy

RENAL SYSTEM:

It is sudden in onset and there is an increased collection of nitrogenous waste in body. Usually, it is reversible.

Aetiology–Decreased I/V fluids in surgical patients results in hypotension which causes acute tubular necrosis.

Treatment–Fluid challenges with 500 cc of normal saline as bolus.

Avoid nephrotoxic drugs in oliguria patients in postoperative period.

G.I. SYSTEM:

Paralytic Ileus – There is a loss of peristalsis, mostly after abdominal surgery. Usually, it lasts from 24 hours to 7 days. Small bowel motility usually comes after 12 to 48 hours. Gastric motility takes 36 to 48 hours. Colonic motility starts after 3 to 7 days.

S/S—Nausea, vomiting and abdominal distension.

Treatment:

- Nil orally and Ryle's tube aspiration
- I/V fluids and electrolyte balance
- Mechanical obstruction to be ruled out

Even in prolonged ileus with no mechanical obstruction, 100 ml of water soluble contrast medium can administered through the tube and X-rays are taken at 15 minutes and 1 hour interval. If contrast is visible in the upper jejunum or beyond, then remove the nasogastric tube and start orally.

Prolonged paralytic ileus (due to increased sympathetic activity) can be treated with Guanethidine.

How to administer: The patient is placed supine. Blood pressure should be normal. 20 mg of Injection

Guanethidine in 100 ml of saline is infused over a period of 40 minutes. B.P. is checked at 10-minute intervals, if it falls below 90 mm Hg systolic, stop infusion immediately. Usually, at the end of the infusion the patient passes flatus and watery stool.

If less dramatic effect with Guanethidine, then give 0.25 ml of Prostigmine I/V over 1 minute and repeat this after 10 minutes.

> Most of the intestinal gas (>70%) is secondary to swallowed air. Flatus generally indicates transit of air from stomach to the anal canal and suggests return of bowel function.

Surgical infections in postoperative period:

For surgical infection, > 1000 colony forming units of virulent bacteria is adequate to colonize a wound but 105 bacteria/mm 3 on tissue culture suggests an established infection. The bacteria needs either blood, necrotic tissue or seroma to thrive.

Examine the patient daily for signs and symptoms of infection:

Local:

- Pain
- Redness
- Temperature
- Oedema
- Loss of function

Systemic:

- Fever

- Chills

- Tachycardia

- Tachypnoea

- Leukocytosis

Increasing pain, erythema, cellulitis or the presence of purulent discharge from the incision indicates that the wound is infected.

If the onset of the infection is within the first 24 hours then it is streptococcus or clostridium.

If it is in 3–4 days then it is postoperative-staphylococcus

Management:

- Drainage

- Debridement

- Drugs (antibiotics)

Common organisms responsible for postoperative local/ systemic infection:

- Gram-Positive cocci

- Staphylococcus Aureus - usually found in infected incisions and at central line

  Treatment: Penicillin, Cephalosporin, Macrolide and Vancomycin

- Streptococcus Faecalis (Enterococcus) - found in all intra-abdominal infections including biliary tract and also in the urinary tract.

  Treatment: Penicillin + Aminoglycosides (e.g. Ampicillin + Gentamicin)

- Streptococcus Pyogenes - found in infected incision

  Treatment: Penicillin G, Erythromycin

- Streptococcus Pneumonaie - causes post-operative pneumonitis

  Treatment: Penicillin G, Erythromycin, Ciprofloxacin

GRAM-POSITIVE BACILLI

- Clostridium Perfringens - causes gas gangrene in POP (post-operative period)

  Treatment: Penicillin

  > If any patient requires more than the required dose of painkillers for wound infection, then they should be suspected of contracting clostridial infection.

GRAM-NEGATIVE COCCI

- Hemophilus Influenzae - causes POP pneumonia

  Treatment: Penicillin

GRAM-NEGATIVE BACILLI

E coli, Klebsiella, Proteus species - cause intra-abdominal infection, wound abscess, UTI, and nosocomial pneumonia

Treatment: Third generation Cephalosporin, Ampicillin

MANAGEMENT OF WOUND INFECTION

Remove the infected suture from the skin, open and drain the wound and send for culture and sensitivities. Examine the underlying fascia for integrity. Change the dressing twice or thrice a day. If healthy granulation tissue is formed, secondary suturing can be done.

If the whole incision is infected, then wound dehiscence can occur. It can be superficial, involving non-healing of skin and subcutaneous tissue, or complete wound dehiscence. Complete wound dehiscence can be due to - infection, ischemia, increased intra-abdominal pressure due to excessive coughing in POP, or due to poor suturing technique.

Treatment:

For superficial dehiscence - dressing thrice a day

For complete dehiscence - wound exploration, debridement, and tensionless resuturing under general anaesthesia, with third generation Cephalosporin + Metronidazole

CAUSES OF POSTOPERATIVE (POP) FEVER

0–2nd POP day

- Atelectasis
- Wound infection with clostridium or streptococcus
- Aspiration pneumonia

3–6th POP day

- UTI - remove catheter if possible
- Wound infection
- Leakage of bowel anastomosis
- IV sites phlebitis (peripheral IV sites should be changed every third day)
- Central venous catheter- remove catheter, if fever settles. No antibiotics

6–10th POP day

- Intra-abdominal abscesses
- Deep vein thrombosis
- Pelvic abscess
- Sinusitis due to prolonged use of nasogastric tube
- Drug fever

PSYCHOLOGICAL COMPLICATIONS IN POP PERIOD

- Hyper arousal
- Confusion and Depression

• Delirium/tremors

Treatment - I/V Injection Chlormethiazole Edisylate, 0.8% infusion. 3–5 ml/minute is given until patient begins to relax.

Take Home Message

1. Prevent complication such as Infection.

2. Promote healing of surgical Wound.

3. Return the patient to a state of health as early as possible.

REFERENCE

1. Kron I L, Harman P K, Nolan S P. The measurement of intra-abdominal pressure as a criterion for abdominal re-exploration. Ann Surg. (1984);199:28–30.

2. Sugrue M, Jones F, Lee A. et al. Intra-abdominal pressure and gastric intramucosal pH: is there an association? W J Surg. (1996);20:988–991.

3. Ivatury R R, Simon R J, Islam S. et al. Intra-abdominal hypertension, gastric mucosal pH and the abdominal compartment syndrome (abstract) J Trauma. (1997);43:194

4. Saggi BH, Sugerman HJ, Ivatury RR, Bloomfield GL. Abdominal compartment syndrome. J Trauma 1998; 45: 597–609.

5. Iberti T J, Kelly K M, Gentili D R. et al. A simple technique to accurately determine

intra-abdominal pressure. Crit Care Med. (1987);15:1140–1142.

6. Ridings P C, Blocher C R, Sugerman H J. Cardiopulmonary effects of raised intra-abdominal pressure before and after intravascular volume expansion. J Trauma. (1995);39:1071–1075.

Chapter 10

ACUTE ABDOMEN

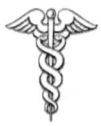

Sunder Goyal

The term acute abdomen refers to a sudden, severe abdominal pain of unclear aetiology. Acute abdomen means when surgery is done in an emergency. Abdomen is a magic box and all abdominal emergencies are challenging. Acute abdomen can occur due to infection (peritonitis), or can be due to ischemia of gut.

Causes of Acute Abdomen-

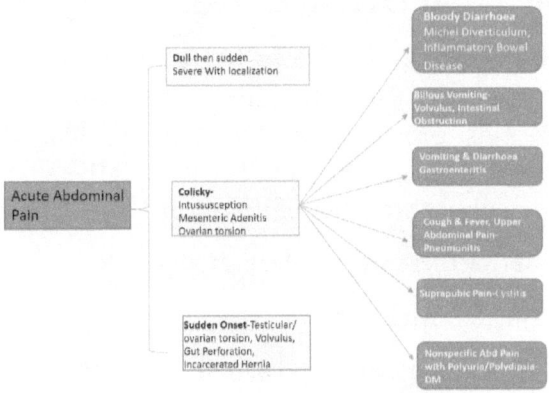

Infants	Child	Adolescent
Intussusception	Appendicitis	Trauma
Incarcerated hernia	Intussusception	Appendicitis
Volvulus	Incarcerated hernia	Ectopic Pregnancy
Appendicitis	Trauma	Testicular/ ovarian Torsion
	Testicular torsion	

INFECTION

Infections result in the inflammation of the peritoneum (peritonitis). On physical examination, there is pain upon removal of pressure more than on the application of pressure to the abdomen (rebound tenderness), and the most specific finding is rigidity.

ISCHEMIC ACUTE ABDOMEN

Vascular disorders are more likely to affect the small bowel than the large bowel. Arterial supply to the intestines is provided by the superior and inferior mesenteric arteries (SMA and IMA respectively), both of which are direct branches of the aorta.

The superior mesenteric artery supplies:

1. Small bowel

2. Ascending and proximal two-thirds of the transverse colon

The inferior mesenteric artery supplies:

1. Distal one-third of the transverse colon

2. Descending colon

3. Sigmoid colon

The splenic flexure (watershed area), the junction between the transverse and descending colon, is supplied by the most distal portions of both the inferior mesenteric artery and superior mesenteric artery, and is always susceptible to ischemia.

Condition causing ischemia of gut:

1. Occlusive Ischemia - A thromboembolism from the left side of the heart resulting in an occlusion of the SMA, such as during atrial fibrillation.

2. Nonocclusive ischemia - In hypotension secondary to cardiac failure. It usually results in a mucosal or mural infarct, whereas thromboembolism of the SMA causes the typically transmural infarct.

3. Hyper coagulable state of blood (in polycythaemia vera) may cause the thrombosis of the primary mesenteric vein resulting in ischemic acute abdomen.

A few medical causes of acute abdomen are:

1. Diabetic ketoacidosis

2. Sickle cell anaemia

3. Adrenal crisis

4. Familial Mediterranean fever

Various surgical causes are:

1. Traumatic–Close/Open----Crush injuries, Stab injuries, Compressing injuries with gut perforation or with massive intraperitoneal bleeding

2. Infections–Appendicitis, Abdominal Abscess, Duodenal Perforation

3. Bleeding–Gastro-intestinal bleeding

4. Vascular Occlusion–Mesenteric vessels

5. Bowel Obstruction

   a. Congenital Causes

   b. Inflammatory Causes

   c. Mechanical Causes

   d. Malignancies

SYMPTOMS OF ACUTE ABDOMEN

These present with diffuse abdominal pain, bowel distention, and bloody diarrhoea.

- Pain – Severity/Radiation/Nature (aggravating and relieving factors)

- VOMITING – Frequency/Character/Colour/Odour

- Distention Abdomen – Whole Abdomen (Upper or Lower).

- Constipation

EXAMINATION

Inspection – Decreased movement of all segments

Visible peristalsis/Visibly enlarged veins

Examine hernial sites for swelling

Palpation/Percussion – Tenderness usually present

Guarding/Rigidity always present

Auscultation— Absent bowel sounds

Rectal/Vaginal Examination is a MUST. Look for tenderness, bogginess and blood on the fingertip.

INVESTIGATIONS

Blood Investigation – A neutrophilic leukocytosis, sometimes with a left shift and raised serum amylase

- X-Ray abdomen (in standing position)
- FAST U/S or/and C.T. Abdomen (if patient is haemodynamically stable)
- Peritoneal tap/lavage
- Diagnostic Laparoscopy

Use of deep sedatives or strong analgesics like opiates can mask the clinical picture in acute abdomen cases, so they should be avoided before the initial clinical examination. However, few studies did not agree and showed that they did not alter the results.

Decision Making:

Firstly examine whether the patient needs surgery or not. The next question is when to operate.

Where minutes count and delay increases morbidity/ mortality (Golden Hour):

- Massive intra peritoneal haemorrhage due to splenic rupture, liver injury, ruptured tubal pregnancy, ruptured mesentery and aneurysm.

Where hours count and delay increases morbidity/mortality:

- Intussusception in infancy
- Strangulation of bowel
- Arterial embolism of mesentery
- Duodenal/gastric perforation
- Perforation of Appendix/Acute appendicitis
- Bowel perforation/Gall bladder perforation

When a delay of more than 12 hours increases morbidity/ mortality:

- Small bowel obstruction
- Volvulus of large gut

Acute emergency, but no surgery is needed:

- Acute pancreatitis
- Regional ileitis
- Mesenteric lymphadenitis
- Acute salpingitis

DEFINITE INDICATION FOR ABDOMINAL SURGERY

It is very important to distinguish true acute abdomen that requires urgent surgical intervention and which can initially be managed conservatively, from those that do not.

1. Persistent pain and guarding–not relieved by painkillers and sedation.

2. Progressive increase in abdominal distention

3. Persistent shock, High grade fever and persistent vomiting

Definite investigations support:

1. Plain X-Ray Abdomen in Standing/Lt lateral decubitus position to see air under diaphragm (80–85 % reliable)

2. FAST U/S Abdomen for fluid/blood in abdomen. (85% reliable)

3. Computerized Tomography in haemodynamically stable patients

4. Paracentesis/peritoneal lavage–Blood > than 5 ml and intestinal fluid where vegetative is positive (90% reliable)

5. Diagnostic Laparoscopy/Mini-Lap—(100% reliable)

DIFFERENTIAL DIAGNOSIS

1. EPIGASTRIC PAIN

   a. Acute gastritis

   b. Acute pancreatitis

   c. Perforated gastric ulcer

2. Right Hypochondrium

   a. Acute cholecystitis

   b. Amoebic liver abscess

   c. Perforated duodenal ulcer

3. Right and Left Lumbar Region

   - Acute renal colic

   - Perinephric abscess

   - Colitis/diverticulitis

   - Perforated diverticulum

4. Right Iliac fossa, Lt. Iliac fossa

   - Appendicitis

   - Acute Typhlitis (Caecal Amoebic infection)

   - Caecal Volvulus/Perforation

   - Acute Salpingitis

   - Meckel's Diverticulum

   - Ruptured Ectopic pregnancy

   - Sigmoid Volvulus

   - Twisted Ovarian cyst

Central area:

Acute Intestinal Obstruction

Mesenteric Artery/Vein Occlusion

Take Home Message

1. Challenge to Surgeons.

2. Commonest cause of surgical emergency admission.

3. Clinical course can vary from minutes to hours, to weeks.

REFERENCES

1. *Walter Siegenthaler (21 March 2007).* Differential diagnosis in internal medicine: from symptom to diagnosis. *Thieme. pp. 257–.* ISBN 978-1-58890-551-2. Retrieved 28 July 2010.

2. Manterola C, Astudillo P, Losada H, Pineda V, Sanhueza A, Vial M (2007). Manterola C, ed. "Analgesia in patients with acute abdominal pain". Cochrane Database Syst Rev (3): CD005660. doi:10.1002/14651858.CD005660.pub2. PMID 17636812.

3. Ranji SR, Goldman LE, Simel DL, Shojania KG (October 2006). "Do opiates affect the clinical evaluation of patients with acute abdominal pain?". JAMA. **296** (14): 1764–74.doi:10.1001/jama.296.14.1764. PMID 17032990.

4. *Scaglione, Mariano; Linsenmaier, Ulrich; Schueller, Gerd (2012).* Emergency Radiology of the Abdomen: Imaging Features and Differential Diagnosis for a Timely Management

Approach. *Springer Science & Business Media. p. 2.* ISBN 9788847025134.

PEPTIC PERFORATION

Peptic ulcer disease (PUD), also known as a peptic ulcer or stomach ulcer, is a break in the lining of the stomach, first part of the small intestine, or occasionally the lower oesophagus.

GASTRIC/DUODENAL PERFORATION

Gastric Ulcer Disease

History: common in elderly/people living in poor socioeconomic conditions

History of burning epigastrium relieved by food

History of chronic alcoholism

History of eating of excessive chilies, mainly red

History of chronic smoking

History of long term use of drugs like Aspirin/ NSAIDS

Usually these patient have hypochlorhydria = less acid secretion

Excessive acid secretions

Common Site of Ulceration

Most common – Anterior surface

The second most common site is Anterior-Superior surface of lesser curvature

Initially – chemical peritonitis due to acid

Infected by bacteria

Pyogenic peritonitis

Symptoms And Signs

- Sudden pain in epigastrium
- Guarding/Rigidity
- Dull abdomen on percussion
- Absent bowel sounds

Investigations

Routine: Haemoglobin, Total and differential leucocytes count

Specific: Erect X-Ray Abdomen in standing position including both domes of diaphragm to see air under diaphragm. (Put 50 – 100 cc air through Ryle's tube and repeat X-Ray if the first X-ray film is negative.)

U/S - 80 to 90 % +ve for fluids in abdomen

Paracentesis (Abdominal tapping):

Management

Ryle's Tube

IV drip

Antibiotics

Urgent surgery - delay is harmful to the patient

Operative Procedure

Upper mid line incision:

Thorough peritoneal toilet with saline is important to decrease the morbidity.

Always use two drains : One in pelvis; One near suture line in right subcostal region

Removal of drain - usually in 5–7 days (when drainage stops).

In the case of severe peritonitis, drain the abdominal wall suture line also to decrease the incidence of wound infection.

Single layer suturing with prolene no. 1 suture including the peritoneum and rectus sheath while suturing. The needle displaces the lateral aspect of cut belly of rectus muscle. So only the peritoneum and the sheath are sutured together.

Interrupted sutures are inserted 1.5 cm away from the wound edge at intervals of 1 cm.

Rectus muscle may or may not be picked up in midline incision while suturing the wound.

Postoperative Care

- Ryle's Tube aspiration is the lifeline
- Ryle's Tube should be maintained till the patient passes flatus - usually 3–5 days/or aspirate in about 200–300/24 hours.

- Antibiotics

- Antacids

- Fluids

- Abdominal drains for 5–7 days

- Usually most patients do not require vagotomy

- Postoperative medical treatment mostly heals the ulcer

- Only 1/3 cases may need vagotomy and/or drainage procedures

- Gastric ulcer may be malignant, so take a biopsy from margin

- Posterior wall ulcer - usually there are more chances of haemorrhage

- If very big ulcer – Gastrectomy Billroth I/I required.

- Laparoscopy - can be managed by using intracorporal suturing or placement. Or through fibrin glue, gelatine sponge or omental patch

  ➢ Chest physiotherapy is very important

  ➢ Early mobilization in postoperative period to avoid deep vein thrombosis

References

1. ajm, WI (September 2011). "Peptic ulcer disease.". Primary care. **38** (3): 383–94, vii. doi:10.1016/j.pop.2011.05.001. PMID 21872087.

2. "Definition and Facts for Peptic Ulcer Disease". National Institute of Diabetes and Digestive and Kidney Diseases. Retrieved 28 February 2015

DUODENAL ULCER

- Duodenal ulcers are rarely malignant
- Major cause is increased acid production
- Recently role of Helicobacter Pylori : Breath test to diagnosis and treatment is-

Cap Amoxicillin 500 mgs TDS +Tab Metrogyl 500 mgs TDS

Both for one week.

Follow the same diagnostic and investigation procedures as for gastric ulcer.

Management

Simple closure with interrupted 0-catgut.

Suture with omental patch (Graham patch).

Due to availability of H_2 receptors antagonist and other anti-ulcer regime – no need of vagotomy, etc.

Proton pump inhibitors – antacids are effective medical treatment.

About 2/3 of such patients become symptom free with medical treatment.

Definite treatment is required for patients where medical treatment fails and there is there is a recurrence of dyspepsia, etc.

Postoperative Complications

Rarely – duodenal fistula

Haemorrhage

Intra-abdominal abscess

References

1. ajm, WI (September 2011). "Peptic ulcer disease.". Primary care. **38** (3): 383–94, vii. doi:10.1016/j.pop.2011.05.001. PMID 21872087.

2. "Definition and Facts for Peptic Ulcer Disease". National Institute of Diabetes and Digestive and Kidney Diseases. Retrieved 28 February 2015

ACUTE APPENDICITIS

These are the most common surgical emergencies

1. Acute Appendicitis

2. Sub-Acute Appendicitis

3. Chronic Appendicitis

4. Recurrent Appendicitis

5. Non-Obstructive Appendicitis

Acute appendicitis: It is a condition in which there is a sudden inflammation of the appendix. The lumen of appendix gets obstructed which causes an invasion of the appendix wall by the gut flora. This condition occurs in the age group of 20–30. Incidence is equal in both sexes, but is more commonly seen among teenage girls.

Sub-Acute Appendicitis: If the episode of acute appendicitis subsides spontaneously before reaching the acute stage, then it is sub-acute appendicitis. This is probably a recurrent condition.

Chronic Appendicitis: Acute inflammation turns into chronic appendicitis. Patients usually present with persistent right lower abdominal pain.

Recurrent Appendicitis: Recurrent appendicitis is not full-blown, acute appendicitis but mild, recurrent attacks. The patients are symptom-free in between.

Non-Obstructive Appendicitis: This is a non-obstructing inflammation of the appendix. There is localized peritonitis. Such an inflammation usually terminates either by gangrene, fibrosis suppuration, or resolution.

Causes and Risk Factors of Appendicitis

The exact cause of appendicitis is not entirely clear; however, the two common causes are:

- Obstruction by fecalith causing infection of the appendix.

- Infection, possibly stomach infection, that has travelled to the site of appendix.

Easy diagnosis and prompt Rx leads to no mortality.

History

Shifting pain from epigastrium to umbilicus to right iliac fossa.

Nausea

Vomiting

Fever

Constipation

Physical Signs

Tenderness at McBurney's point

Rigidity/guarding over right iliac fossa

Rovsing sign +ve

Psoas test +ve

Obturator sign +ve

P/R – in case of pelvic position of appendix- P/R is always tender

Lab test. Increased WBC count

Plain Film Abdomen

U/S abdomen (Diagnostic up to 80 %)

Differential Diagnosis

Mesenteric Adenitis

Meckel's Diverticulitis

Crohn's Disease

Omental Torsion

Diverticulitis

Intussusception in children

Lymphomas

Ureteric colic

Salpingitis, Ruptured ectopic, Twisted ovarian

Management

I/V Fluids

  Ryle Tube Aspiration

  Antibiotics

If no mass

Appendicectomy (Open or Laparoscopic)

If mass

Interval appendicectomy (Open or Laparoscopic)

  Rule out appendiceal abscess; if present, then drain extra-peritoneally

Absolute indication of Open Appendectomy: There may be cases where laparoscopic appendectomy is not the recommended procedure and hence traditional appendectomy will be required. A traditional appendectomy leaves a larger scar and has a larger recovery time. Various factors that lead to traditional appendectomy are:

- Cases where the appendix has burst.

- Patients with tumours in their digestive system.

- Women who are in the first trimester of pregnancy.

- Patients who have had repeated previous abdominal surgery.

Complications

Paralytic Ileus

  Wound Infection

Chapter 11

INTESTINAL OBSTRUCTION

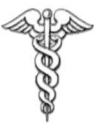

Intestinal obstruction is also known as bowel obstruction. This can be a mechanical or functional obstruction of the intestines which prevents the normal movement of the products of digestion. Obstruction can affect either the small bowel or large bowel.

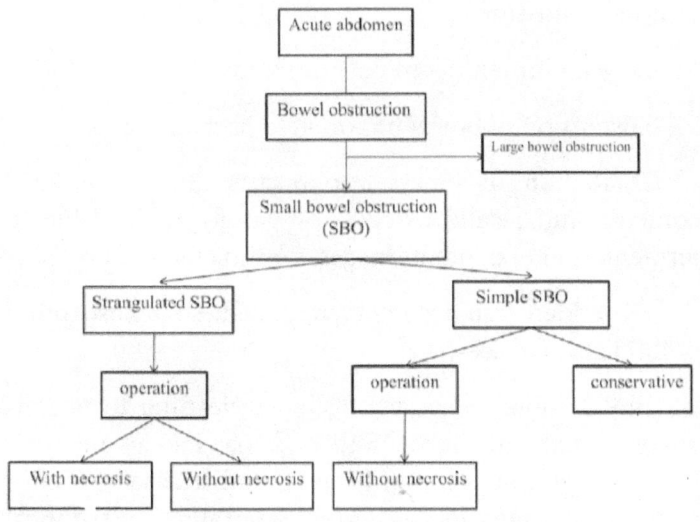

Small Intestine Obstruction

Most common surgical emergency of small intestine

Types

- Complete obstruction

- Incomplete or partial obstruction

It can be dynamic (physical blockage) or

Adynamic-- (stasis of bowel contents)

PATHOPHYSIOLOGY

Dynamic Intestinal Obstruction

Only lumen occlusion

Occlusion of blood supply due to compression leads to gangrene of gut.

Simple occlusion

Pressure on lumen (from outside) leads to--

Distension of bowel proximal to obstruction.

Distention of bowel also occurs due to retained contents and swallowed gas, or gas formation due to fermentation of contents by gas-forming bacteria.

Distended gut becomes congested, so reabsorption of fluid also reduces.

Blood supply also gets occluded, leading to venous engorgement and bowel wall oedema; Patchy neurosis of bowel wall; Invasion of bacteria and release of toxins; Complete gangrene of wall; Perforation; Peritoneal spillage. The infection, may enter circulation via intestinal lymphatics, or go to the circulatory system via direct absorption from the peritoneal wall, leading to SEPTIC SHOCK.

Causes:

Outside the Gut Wall

- Congenital-

    Bands and adhesions

- Inflammatory-

    Previous diverticulitis

Pelvic inflammatory disease

- Traumatic-

    Blunt trauma abdomen

    Adhesions due to previous abdominal surgery

- Malignancy-

    Intra-abdominal malignancies create adhesions

- Hernias

- Volvulus

- Intussusception

WITHIN THE WALL

- Congenital

    Atresia

- Inflammatory

    ➤ Crohn's disease

    ➤ Tuberculosis

- Malignancy

  Carcinoma of gut wall

Adynamic Inst Obstruction

Causes

- Electrolyte imbalance-

  Hypokalaemia

  Hyponatremia

- Metabolic
- Drugs induced:

  Tricyclic anti-depressant drug

  Drugs used for general anaesthesia

- Peritoneal sepsis
- Recent abdominal surgery (postoperative)
- Hypothermia
- Retroperitoneal haemorrhage
- Mesenteric vascular disease
- Diabetic ketoacidosis
- Uraemia

Clinical Features

- Perfuse vomiting
- Abdominal pain

- Progressive abdomen distension

- Higher the obstruction (less distension and more pain)

Signs

- Dehydration – dry tongue

- Fast pulse

- Feeble/absent intestinal sounds

- Tingling sounds i.e. high-pitched sounds may be heard due to displacement of fluid in dilated loop of gut. Rectal examination is very important (Usually ballooning of rectum is present).

Investigation

- TLC-DLC may be high in septic disease

- Electrolyte abnormalities

- Blood Urea, Serum Creatinine may be high due to dehydration

- Blood sugar to rule out diabetes mellitus

- Plain X-Ray abdomen – it is 60 to 80% diagnostic

- X-Ray Abdomen in supine and erect position

It gives all information:

a. Shows air fluid level in stepladder pattern.

b. If dilated, bowel diameter is about 5 cm, it is pathological

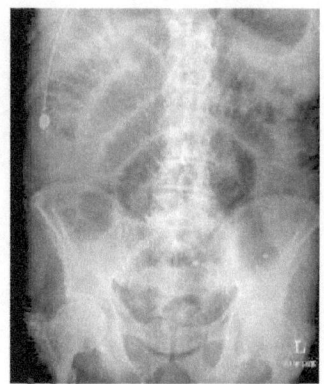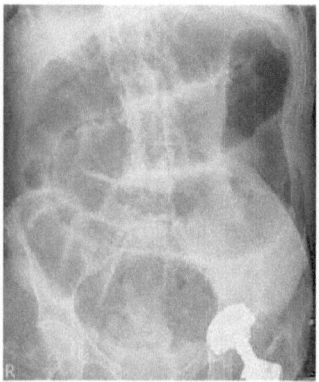

X-Rays-Small bowel and Large bowel obstruction

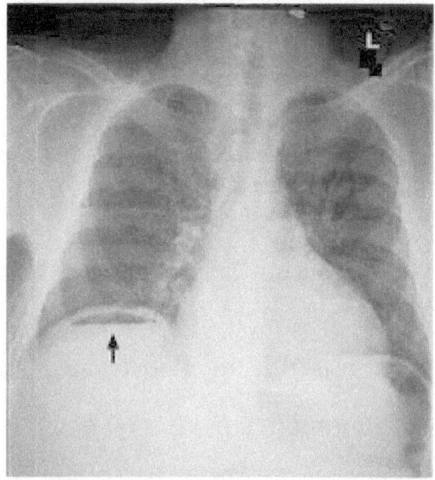

Erect film shows air leakage (air under diaphragm)

- Ultrasound Abdomen

  a. Shows dilated loops. If dilatation is more than 3 cm, it is pathological.

  b. Shows peritoneal fluid due to intestinal leakage

c. Important: In intussusception cases, especially for children, X-rays should be avoided

d. Useful for pregnant patients where radiation is contraindicated.

- Computer Tomography

    Advantage to detect external pressure on small intestine e.g. abscess, haematoma and tumours

Treatment

In the management of small bowel obstructions, a commonly quoted surgical aphorism is: "Never let the sun rise or set on small-bowel obstruction," Because about 5.5% [1] of small bowel obstructions are ultimately fatal, if treatment is delayed.

Nil orally

I/V fluid – NS/RL

Continuous Ryle Tube aspiration as well as intermittent aspiration

Antibiotics

Correction of electrolytes: sodium, potassium, chloride

Catheterize the patient to monitor output and renal functions

When to operate:

If high grade fever persists

Persistent Tachycardia

Increasing distension/tenderness

High TLC/DLC (Rising)

Signs and symptoms of strangulation of gut – septic shock

Operative Management:

Midline incision

Find out the cause of obstruction.

Decompress the obstructed bowel

    a. By needle decompression

    b. Via a small enterotomy

- Abdominal muscle must be relaxed to reduce intra-abdominal pressure and for easy retraction of abdominal wall.

- Avoid catching any bowel loop between wall and retractor.

- Small bowel is a long tube, many meters long. Protect the loop by covering with warm saline mops to avoid drying of gut.

- Pack away the bowel within the abdomen with the help of a large wet gauge pack

- Suction tip may be blocked by solid debris and blood clots. Remove all these with the help of swabs.

- Always counts swabs/instruments when you start closing the abdomen.

- Explore whole gut. Start at duodenojejunal flexure and carry on upwards to the ileocaecal junction, whole length of small bowel and its mesentery.

- Bowel viability

- Colour

- Mobility – peristalsis

- Presence of mesentery arterial pulsation

If gut viability is doubtful – increase oxygen to 100% and cover the gut loop with a warm saline mop.

GUT ANASTOMOSIS

- Both ends should be healthy and viable

- Fresh blood ooze from both ends

- Both openings almost equal size

- No tension

- Single layer (latest)

Two layer (old technique)

Single layer interrupted	Double layer internal continuous
mucosa heals rapidly and water tight formed within 24 hours and heals fast	Outer Seromuscular layer suturing causes narrowing of the lumen with greater tissue strangulation
No narrowing of gut in early phase	Tends to narrow lumen in early phase due to postoperative oedema.

Single layer suturing of end to end, small bowel anastomosis is ideal.

Suture material: 000/00 Vicryl on round body suture is the thread of choice.

Outer layer with 000/00 silk with round body.

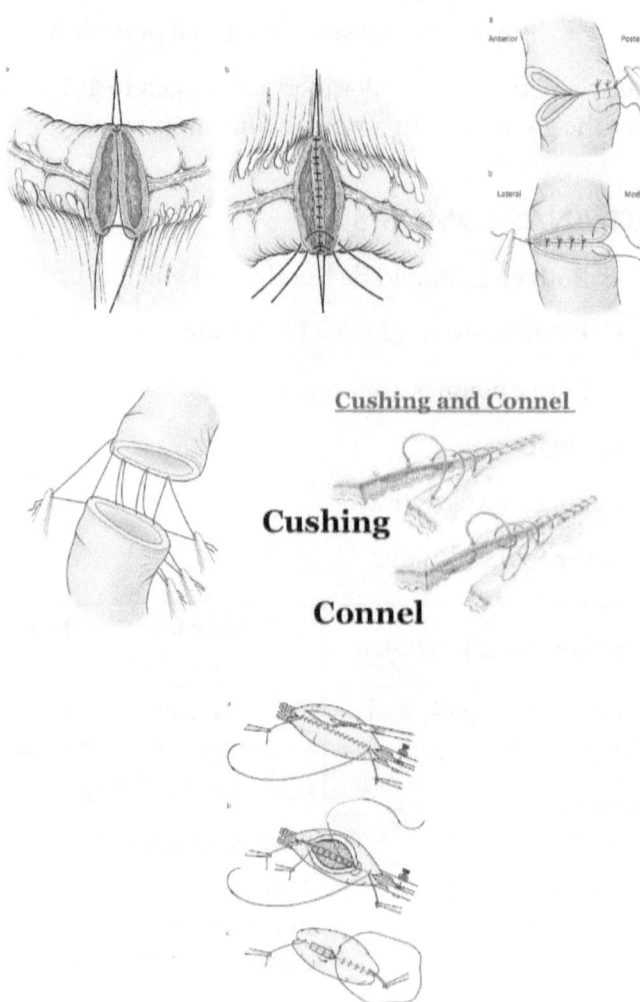

Cushing and Connel

Cushing

Connel

Drains

Usually anastomosis leak after 1–2 weeks, so drain may be kept up to two weeks. But a drain in contact with anastomosis for this length of time could, in itself, cause damage, so drain can be removed after 5–7 days when drainage in tube ceases.

So low pressure drain.

Drain inserted for bleeding - up to 48–72 hrs

Drain inserted for anastomosis leak- up to 5 to 7 days.

Role of mechanical stapling devices within the abdomen:

Mechanical stapling devices have improved the anastomosis technique.

Advantage - Speed.

Useful when access is limited.

Instruments and gloves which have been contaminated during anastomosis should not be used for the closure of the abdominal wall to avoid postoperative wound infection. (Infection can lead to wound dehiscence and incisional hernia).

LARGE GUT OBSTRUCTION

The incidence of this is ten times lower compared to small bowel obstruction.

Morbidity and mortality is higher than small bowel obstruction due to:

- High contents of bacteria in lumen
- More chances of perforation and gangrene

- Signs/symptoms appear slowly

- Mostly in elderly

Causes

- Inflammatory bowel disease

- Malignancies

- Volvulus sigmoid colon

- Volvulus caecum

- Adhesions

- Extensive pressure on lumen

- Faecal impaction and pseudo obstruction

Clinical features

Depending on the basic cause of the obstruction, these vary with primary disease

    a.   along with degree of obstruction

    b.   causes of obstruction

    c.   degree of onset

    d.   ileo-caecal valve competency

    e.   presence of other conditions

Pathophysiology of Large Bowel Obstruction

- Intra luminary pressure is very high in large bowel obstruction as compare to small bowel obstruction.

- Bacteria present in the bowel play an important role in the disease process as organization is very high in number in the large bowel, i.e. coli form and anaerobic.

Signs/symptoms

- Pain

- Vomiting

- Distension of abdomen

- Alteration of bowel habits

- Visible distended loops of gut

- Sometime rigidity/guarding/tenderness

- Shock

- Mass may be palpable in obstruction due to malignancy

  Rectal examination is very important, as is Ryle Tube aspiration

Diagnosis

- Routine Investigations

- TBC (total blood count)

- Electrolytes

- Blood Sugar

- Serum creatinine

- Plain X-ray abdomen in supine and in standing (Plain X-ray abdomen has up to 90% positive sensitivity)

- Ultrasound of Abdomen

- Proctoscopy

- Sigmoidoscopic

- Colonoscopy

- Computed Tomography Scan

Differential Diagnosis

Differential diagnoses of bowel obstruction include:

- Ileus

- Pseudo-obstruction or Ogilvie's syndrome

- Intra-abdominal sepsis

- Pneumonia or other systemic illness

Treatment:

Ryle Tube aspiration

I/V fluids Ringer Lactate/Normal Saline

Broad spectrum antibiotics covering both gram+ and gram-ve bacteria and Bacteroides

Ideally:

Cephalosporin (3rd generation)

Aminoglycoside

Aztreonam (if renal failure)

Metrogyl

Treatment can be

- Conservative

    Treatment for intestinal obstruction depends on the cause of the condition, but generally requires hospitalization.

When the patient arrives at the hospital, first stabilize the patient so that they can undergo definite treatment. This process may include:

- Placing an intravenous (IV) line into a vein so that fluids can be given

- Putting a nasogastric tube to suck out air and fluid from stomach and thus to relieve abdominal swelling

- Placing a catheter into the bladder to drain urine and collect it for testing

TREATING INTUSSUSCEPTION

A barium or air enema is used, both as a diagnostic procedure and as a treatment for children with intussusception. If an enema works, further treatment is usually not necessary.

TREATMENT FOR PARTIAL OBSTRUCTION

If the patient has an obstruction through which some food and fluid can still get through (partial obstruction), he may not need further treatment after being stabilized. Recommend a special low-fibre diet that is easier for the partially blocked intestine to process. If the obstruction does not clear on its own, the patient may need surgery to relieve the obstruction.

TREATMENT FOR COMPLETE OBSTRUCTION

If nothing is able to pass through the intestine, you may recommend surgery to relieve the blockage. The procedure will depend on what's causing the obstruction and which part of the intestine is affected. Surgery typically involves removing the obstruction, as well as any section of the intestine that has died or is damaged.

Alternatively, you may recommend treating the obstruction with a self-expanding metal stent. The wire mesh tube is inserted into the colon via an endoscope passed through the mouth or colon. It forces open the colon so that the obstruction can clear.

Stents are generally used to treat people with colon cancer, or to provide temporary relief in people for whom emergency surgery is too risky. The patient may still need surgery, once his condition is stable.

TREATMENT FOR PSEUDO-OBSTRUCTION

If you determine that the signs and symptoms are caused by pseudo-obstruction (paralytic ileus), monitor the patient's condition for a day or two in the hospital, and treat the cause if it's known. Paralytic ileus can get better on its own. In the meantime, feed the patient through a nasal tube or an IV to prevent malnutrition.

If paralytic ileus doesn't improve on its own, prescribe medication that causes muscle contractions, which can help move food and fluids through the intestines. If paralytic ileus is caused by an illness or medication, then treat the underlying illness or stop the medication. In rare cases, surgery may be needed to remove part of the intestine.

In cases where the colon is enlarged, a treatment called decompression may provide relief. Decompression can be done with colonoscopy, a procedure in which a thin tube is inserted into the anus and guided into the colon. Decompression can also be done through surgery.

- **Operative**

    Preoperative stoma marking for colostomy or ileostomy is very important

    Midline incision

    Decompress the large gut

    Protective colostomy prior to anastomosis

How to do anastomosis:

Single layer with silk is done

In the postoperative period, prevention of deep vein thrombosis is very important, as patients mostly belong to an older age group.

PSEUDO-OBSTRUCTION (PARALYTIC ILEUS)

Here, there is no physical obstruction yet the patient presents with signs and symptoms of intestinal obstruction. In paralytic ileus, muscles or nerve problems disrupt the normal coordinated muscle contractions of the intestines, slowing or stopping the movement of food and fluid through the digestive system. Paralytic ileus can affect any part of the intestine.

Causes can be:

- Abdominal or pelvic surgery

- Infection

- Certain medications that affect muscles and nerves, including tricyclic antidepressants, such as amitriptyline and imipramine (Tofranil), and opioid pain medications, such as those containing hydrocodone (Vicodin) and oxycodone (Oxycontin)

- Muscle and nerve disorders, such as Parkinson's disease

Risk Factors

Diseases and conditions that can increase the risk of intestinal obstruction include:

- Abdominal or pelvic surgery which often causes adhesions — a common intestinal obstruction

- Crohn's disease, which can cause the intestine's walls to thicken, narrowing the passageway

- Cancer in your abdomen, especially if you've had surgery to remove an abdominal tumour or radiation therapy

Complications

Untreated, intestinal obstruction can cause serious, life-threatening complications, including:

- **Tissue death.** Intestinal obstruction can cut off the blood supply to a part of your intestine. Lack of blood causes the intestinal wall to die. Tissue death can result in a tear (perforation) in the intestinal wall, which can lead to infection.

- **Infection.** Peritonitis is the medical term for infection in the abdominal cavity. It's a life-threatening condition that requires immediate medical, and often. surgical attention.

Take Home Message

1. Abdominal pain, distension, vomiting and constipation are four cardinal signs of Intestinal Obstruction.

2. Never miss hernial site examination in Intestinal obstruction.

3. Always correct fluids & electrolytes imbalance and match with lab results in Intestinal Obstruction.

4. Get X-Ray Abdomen in Supine, Erect position along with X-Ray Chest. If patient can't stand for erect film then in decubitus position to see air under diaphragm.

5. Be attentive of signs of peritonitis due to perforation or ischemia of bowel.

6. Always provide adequate resuscitation to the patient.

REFERENCES

1. DD Maglinte; FM Kelvin; MG Rowe MG; GN Bender GN; DM Rouch (January 1, 2001). "Small-bowel obstruction: optimizing radiologic investigation and nonsurgical management". Radiology. 218 (1): 39–46. PMID 11152777.

2. Feldman M, et al. Intestinal obstruction. In: Sleisenger and Fordtran's Gastrointestinal and Liver Disease: Pathophysiology, Diagnosis, Management. 10th ed. Philadelphia, Pa.: Saunders Elsevier;   2016.   http://www.clinicalkey.com. Accessed Sept. 10, 2015.

3. Glancy DG. Intestinal obstruction. Surgery. 2014;34:204.

4. Kitagawa S, et al. Intussusception in children. http://www.uptodate.com/home. Accessed Sept. 10, 2015.

5. Intestinal pseudo-obstruction. National Institute of Diabetes and Digestive and Kidney Diseases http://www.niddk.nih.gov/health-information/ health-topics/digestive-diseases/intestinal-pseudo-obstruction/Pages/facts.aspx.   Accessed Sept. 17, 2015.

6. *Gore, RM; Silvers, RI; Thakrar, KH; Wenzke, DR; Mehta, UK; Newmark, GM; Berlin, JW (November 2015). "Bowel Obstruction.". Radiologic clinics of North America. 53 (6): 1225 40.* PMID 26526435. doi:10.1016/j.rcl.2015.06.008.

7. *Fitzgerald, J. Edward F. (2010).* Small Bowel Obstruction. *Oxford:* Wiley-Blackwell *pp. 74*

8. ISBN 9781405170253. doi:10.1002/9781444315172. ch14. Archived *from the original on September 8, 2017.*

VOLVULUS CAECUM

Less common than sigmoid volvulus

Causes

- Underlying failure of fixation of ileal and caecal mesentery to the posterior abdominal wall

- Increased chances during pregnancy

- After abdominal surgeries

- In patient with distal colonic obstruction

Clinical Features

- Vomiting

- Colicky pain

- Abdominal distension

- Palpable mass in splenic area

- Empty right iliac fossa

- Volvulus rotation is in clockwise direction

- Age group – 40 to 60 years

- Incidence about 2% of total intestinal obstruction

Diagnosis

- Plain X-ray Abdomen +ve in 90% of cases

- Comma shaped caecal shadow in mid abdomen or upper left quadrant with concavity facing the right iliac fossa

- Erect film shows a single fluid level

- If caecal perforation, then gas under diaphragm

- A water soluble contract enema produces tapered narrowing in ascending colon

Management

General:

- Ryle's Tube Aspiration

- I/V fluids

- Antibiotics

Specific:

Early intervention is a must as caecal perforation is common

Colonoscopy may be attempted

Midline incision is used

Decompress the tense caecum with needle suction

Untwist by anti-clock wise rotation

If viable caecum:

- Laparoscopic tube cecostomy

- Coecopaxy cecostomy

If unviable caecum:

- Right hemicolectomy

- Resection with exteriorization

- Resection of caecum and ileocolic anastomosis

SIGMOID VOLVULUS

Incidence is very high - up to 20% of all cases of acute intestinal obstruction

More in males than females

More in poor people

Is related to new wheat season in North India

Age = 45 to 60 years

Sigmoid colon becomes elongated and rotates around narrowed sigmoid mesentery through 180^0–360^0 in either a clockwise or an anticlockwise direction - usually anticlockwise. Usually 10–15 % of patients present late with gangrene gut.

Predisposing Factors

- Absence of the last band of lane

- Narrowing of pedicle of sigmoid colon due to fibrosis

- A wide left paracolic gutter

Clinical Features

- Abdominal pain

- Distension

- Constipation

- If hypotension - think of gangrene

- Tachycardia

- Ischemia and gangrene of gut

- Guarding/rigidity

- Ileo-sigmoid knotting, twist around base of mesocolon and also can turn gangrenous

In 50% of the cases usually H/O previous attack +ve

Visible loop on inspection

Palpation: tender, distended colour

No bowel peristalsis due to paralytic ileus.

Diagnosis

Plain X-ray Abdomen in erect position

Shows bent inner tube (omega size) convexity of loop upward and narrow base (bird's beak sign)

Water soluble contrast enema shows beak of a bird of prey (ace of spade sign)

Treatment

- Trial of nonoperative de-rotation with rectal (flatus) tube or with rigid sigmoidoscope.

- If there is gangrene of loop of sigmoid colon then de-rotation and sigmoid resection with proper anastomosis.

MESO-SIGMOIDOPLASTY

Modified meso-sigmoidoplasty - for viable sigmoid colon. It broadens narrow mesocolon.

Procedure

Lower left paramedian incision

Distended sigmoid loop is delivered and untwisted

The peritoneum over the outer aspect of the meso-colon is incised vertically in the middle, taking care not to damage vessel

Incision is made on the sigmoid peritoneum loop to create a window

Two flaps of peritoneum are raised gently for some distance laterally

Sigmoid colon is deflated with a rectal tube

The vertically raised flaps (window) - is stitched transversely using continued 2–0 catgut/vicryl suture on round small body needle. This shortens the mesocolon and broadens its base. Recurrence rate is 2 to 5 %.

References

Akhrar Munir, Ikramullah Khan. Management of viable sigmoid volvulus by Mesosigmoidoplasty. Gomal Journal of Medical Sciences Jan-June 2009, Vol 7, No 1, page 7–9.

COLORECTAL CANCER

It is quite common in the case of large gut obstruction.

Incidence is 25% of all large gut obstruction.

Management depends up to site of growth.

Acute Idiopathic Colonic Pseudo-Obstruction (Ogilvie Syndrome)

No mechanical cause. It occurs due to imbalance between sympathetic-parasympathetic control of peristalsis in the distal colon.

Predisposing Conditions

Renal failure

Orthopaedic trauma

Electrolyte imbalance

Cerebrovascular accident

Puerperium

Massive myocardial infection

Myxoedema

Clinical Features

Resembles mechanical obstruction

Pain

Vomiting

Distension

Untreated cases may have caecal perforation due to retrograde increased pressure in caecum

Diagnosis

Plain film shows distended large bowel with tail off at the splenic flexure or rectosigmoid region

Contrast shadow is very important to rule out mechanical obstruction

Non-Operative Rx

Medical Rx

Ryle Tube aspiration

I/V fluid

Correction of fluid and electrolyte imbalance

Treatment of predisposing cause

Flatus tube and enema

Epidural Anaesthesia

I/V Guanethidine 20 mg in 200 ml of saline followed by increments of Neostigmine 0.05 mg every 3–4 minutes up to a total 0.5 mg of the drug.

Colonoscopy

Success rate up to 80%

Danger of perforation is more than with rigid colonoscope

Perforation chances are less in flexible colonoscopy

In case of failed colonoscopy due to faecal matter loaded descending colon, CT guided percutaneous retroperitoneal needle (22 gauge) aspiration of air can be done to release back pressure on caecum.

Operative Treatment

Indication: if there are signs of impending caecal rupture

If diameter of caecum approaches up to 12 cm or more with patent ileo-caecal valve, then proceed with cecostomy under LA/A. Wide hole cecostomy instead of tube cecostomy is recommended, as there are more chances of blockage with tube cecostomy.

[Jeffrey R. Crass, Richard L. Simmons, Mathis P. Frick, and Charles W. Maile. **Percutaneous Decompression of the Colon Using CT Guidance in Ogilvie Syndrome. AJR:144, March 1985, page 475–476.**]

Chapter 12

EMERGENCY LAPAROTOMY FOR PERITONEAL INFECTION

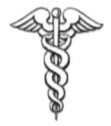

Soiling of peritoneal cavity with perforated hollow viscous results in peritonitis. Injury can be blunt trauma or perforating.

Standard infecting organisms are aerobes and anaerobes - mainly E. Coli and B fragilis. Large gut soiling is more dangerous as infective contents in gut are very high.

CLINICAL PICTURE

Vomiting

High fever with rigors and chills

Abdominal pain

Pulse 100 to 140/mt

Shallow respiration

Low blood pressure

On examination:

Tender drum-like abdomen

Rigidity and rebound tenderness present

Diagnosis

History and clinical picture suggest peritonitis

High TLC/DLC count

X-Ray Abdomen in standing position - air and fluid levels

Air under diaphragm may be there

Soft tissue mass may be displacing adjacent bowel or other organs

In case of sub-diaphragmatic abscess, sympathetic plural effusion

Lung atelectasis (lower lobe)

Ultrasound:

Ultra-sonography is very, very effective. It tells you the location site of collection, character and amount of collection,

CT Scan:

It is also an extremely sensitive modality but CT appearances are non-specific. You get better results with oval contrast.

Management

Ryle tube aspiration:

I/V fluids

Broad spectrum antibiotics like 3rd generation Cephalosporin. Injection Metrogyl

Peritoneal Drainage:

For liver and localised abscess ultrasonography or CT guided aspiration is done and up to 90% is success rate

Contraindicated for needle aspiration:

Ill-defined, not well-formed abscess

Inter loop abscess

Necrotic tumour mass as it will spread along the track to skin

Fungal abscess

Open surgical drainage:

If abscess is poorly defined or difficult to localize by U/S or CT

Very thick, tenacious abscess where needle aspiration fails

The approach entails perforation of a hollow viscous

For generalized peritonitis:

Midline incision

Peritoneal lavage

Drainage

Wound management is very important as wound is very much prone to infection.

Postoperative residual abscess may result in:

Sub-phrenic/sub-hepatic abscess

Paracolic abscess

Splenic abscess

Intra loop abscess

Peritonitis is defined as an inflammation of the serosal membrane that lines the abdominal cavity and the organs contained therein. The peritonitis is mostly infectious but may be sterile (i.e., chemical or mechanical).[1]

Peritoneal infections are classified as Primary (i.e., from hematogenous dissemination, usually in the setting of an immunocompromised state). Primary peritonitis is most often spontaneous bacterial peritonitis (SBP) seen mostly in patients with chronic liver disease.

Secondary (i.e., related to a pathologic process in a visceral organ, such as perforation or trauma, including iatrogenic trauma), or tertiary (i.e., persistent or recurrent infection after adequate initial therapy).

Secondary peritonitis is by far the most common form of peritonitis encountered in clinical practice.

Tertiary peritonitis often develops in the absence of the original visceral organ pathology.

PATHOPHYSIOLOGY

In peritonitis caused by bacteria, the physiologic response depends upon many factors, including the virulence of the contaminant, the size of the inoculum, the immune status and overall health of the host (e.g., as indicated by the Acute Physiology and Chronic Health Evaluation II [APACHE II] score), and elements of the local environment, such as necrotic tissue, blood, or bile.[2]

Intra-abdominal sepsis from a perforated viscus (i.e., secondary peritonitis or suppurative peritonitis) results from direct spillage of luminal contents into the peritoneum (e.g., perforated peptic ulcer, diverticulitis, appendicitis, iatrogenic perforation). With the spillage of the contents, gram-negative and anaerobic bacteria, including common gut flora, such as *Escherichia coli* and *Klebsiella pneumoniae*, enter the peritoneal cavity. Endotoxins produced by gram-negative bacteria lead to the release of cytokines that induce cellular and humoral cascades, resulting in cellular damage, septic shock, and multiple organ dysfunction syndrome (MODS).

The mechanism for bacterial inoculation of ascites has been the subject of much debate since Harold Conn first recognized it in the 1960s. Enteric organisms have traditionally been isolated from more than 90% of infected ascites fluid in spontaneous bacterial peritonitis (SBP), suggesting that the GI tract is the source of bacterial contamination. The preponderance of enteric organisms, in combination with the presence of endotoxin in ascitic fluid and blood, once favoured the argument that SBP was due to direct transmural migration of bacteria from an intestinal or hollow organ lumen, a phenomenon called bacterial translocation. However, experimental evidence suggests that direct transmural migration of microorganisms might not be the cause of SBP.

An alternative proposed mechanism for bacterial inoculation of ascites suggests a hematogenous source of the infecting organism in combination with an impaired immune defence system. Nonetheless, the exact mechanism of bacterial displacement from the GI tract into ascites fluid remains the source of much debate.

A host of factors contributes to the formation of peritoneal inflammation and bacterial growth in the ascitic fluid. A key predisposing factor may be the intestinal bacterial overgrowth found in people with cirrhosis, mainly attributed to decreased intestinal transit time. Intestinal bacterial overgrowth, along with impaired phagocytic function, low serum and ascites complement levels, and decreased activity of the reticuloendothelial system, contributes to an increased number of microorganisms and decreased capacity to clear them from the bloodstream, resulting in their migration into and eventual proliferation within ascites fluid.

Interestingly, adults with SBP typically have ascites, but most children with SBP do not have ascites. The reason for and the mechanism behind this is the source of ongoing investigation.

BACTERIAL LOAD

Bacterial load and the nature of the pathogen also play important roles. The bacterial load may overwhelm the local host defence.

BACTERIAL VIRULENCE

Bacterial virulence factors[3] that interfere with phagocytosis and result in abscess formation. Interaction between certain bacterial and fungal organisms may also play an important role in harming the host's defence. One such synergy may exist between *Bacteroides fragilis* and gram-negative bacteria, particularly *E coli*), where co-inoculation significantly increases bacterial proliferation and abscess formation.

FUNGI

The role of fungi in the formation of intra-abdominal abscesses is not fully understood. Some authors suggest that bacteria and fungi exist as non-synergistic parallel infections with incomplete competition, allowing the survival of all organisms. In this setting, treatment of the bacterial infection alone may lead to an overgrowth of fungi, which may contribute to increased morbidity.

ABSCESS FORMATION

Abscess formation occurs when the host's defence is unable to eliminate the infecting agent and attempts to control the spread of this agent by compartmentalization. This process is aided by a combination of factors that share a common feature, i.e., impairment of phagocytotic killing. Most animal and human studies suggest that abscess formation occurs only in the presence of abscess-potentiating agents. Although the nature and spectrum of these factors have not been studied exhaustively, certain fibre analogues (e.g., bran) and the contents of autoclaved stool have been identified as abscess-potentiating agents. In animal models, these factors inhibit opsonization and phagocytotic killing by interfering with complement activation.

AETIOLOGY

Type	Definition	Microbiology
Table 1 **Classification of peritonitis**		
Primary	A peritoneal infection developing in the absence of a break in the integrity of the gastrointestinal tract, as a result of hematogenous or lymphatic seeding, or bacterial translocation	Monomicrobial infection due to gram-negative *Enterobacteriaceae* or streptococci
Secondary	A peritoneal infection developing in conjunction with an inflammatory process of the gastrointestinal tract or its extensions, usually associated with microscopic or macroscopic perforation	Polymicrobial infection due to aerobic gram-negative bacilli, gram-positive cocci, and enteric anaerobes
Tertiary	A persistent or recurrent peritoneal infection developing after initial treatment of secondary peritonitis	Nosocomial organisms, including resistant gram negative-bacilli, enterococci, staphylococci, and yeast

The aetiology of disease depends on the type, as well as the location, of peritonitis, as follows:

- Primary peritonitis
- Secondary peritonitis
- Tertiary peritonitis
- Chemical peritonitis
- Peritoneal abscess

Primary Peritonitis

Spontaneous bacterial peritonitis (SBP) is an acute bacterial infection of ascitic fluid. Contamination of the peritoneal cavity is thought to result from the translocation of bacteria across the gut wall or mesenteric lymphatics and, less frequently, via hematogenous seeding in the presence of bacteraemia.

Secondary Peritonitis

Common etiologic entities of secondary peritonitis (SP) include perforated appendicitis; perforated gastric or duodenal ulcer; perforated (sigmoid) colon caused by diverticulitis, volvulus, or cancer; and strangulation of the small bowel. Necrotizing pancreatitis can also be associated with peritonitis in the case of infection of the necrotic tissue.

Other rare, nonsurgical causes of intra-abdominal sepsis include the following:

- *Chlamydia* peritonitis

- Tuberculosis peritonitis

- Acquired immunodeficiency syndrome (AIDS)-associated peritonitis

The most common cause of postoperative peritonitis is anastomotic leak, with symptoms generally appearing around postoperative days 5–7. After elective abdominal operations for non-infectious aetiologies, the incidence of secondary peritonitis (SP) (caused by anastomotic disruption, breakdown of enterotomy closures, or inadvertent bowel injury) should be less than 2%. Operations for inflammatory disease (i.e., appendicitis, diverticulitis, cholecystitis) without perforation, carry a risk of less than 10% for the development of SP and peritoneal abscess. This risk may rise to greater than 50% in gangrenous bowel disease and visceral perforation.

After surgeries for penetrating abdominal trauma, SP and abscess formation are observed in a small number of patients. Duodenal and pancreatic involvement, as well as colon perforation, gross peritoneal contamination, perioperative shock and massive transfusion are factors that increase the risk of infection in these cases.

Peritonitis is also a frequent complication and significant limitation of peritoneal dialysis. [3] Peritonitis leads to increased hospitalization and mortality rates.

Tertiary Peritonitis

Tertiary peritonitis develops more frequently in immunocompromised patients and in persons with significant pre-existing, comorbid conditions. Although rarely observed in uncomplicated peritoneal infections, the incidence of tertiary peritonitis in patients requiring ICU admission for severe abdominal infections may be as high as 50–74%.

Gram-positive	*Staphylococcus* species
Fungal	*Candida* species

Peritoneal Abscess

Peritoneal abscess describes the formation of an infected fluid collection encapsulated by fibrinous exudate, omentum, and/or adjacent visceral organs. The overwhelming majority of abscesses occur subsequent to SP. Abscess formation may be a complication of surgery. The incidence of abscess formation after abdominal surgery is less than 1–2%, even when the operation is performed for an acute inflammatory process. The risk of abscess increases to 10–30% in cases of preoperative perforation of the hollow viscus, significant faecal contamination of the peritoneal cavity, bowel ischemia, delayed diagnosis and therapy of the initial peritonitis, and the need for reoperation, as well as in the setting of immunosuppression. Abscess formation is the leading cause of persistent infection and development of tertiary peritonitis.

Prognosis

Over the past decade, the combination of better antibiotic therapy, more aggressive intensive care, and earlier diagnosis and therapy with a combination of operative and percutaneous techniques have led to a significant reduction in morbidity and mortality related to intra-abdominal sepsis.

REFERENCES

1. Pavlidis TE. Cellular changes in association with defence mechanisms in intra-abdominal sepsis. Minerva Chir. 2003 Dec. 58(6):777-81. [Medline].

2. Appenrodt B, Grunhage F, Gentemann MG, Thyssen L, Sauerbruch T, Lammert F. Nucleotide-binding oligomerization domain containing 2 (NOD2) variants are genetic risk factors for death and spontaneous bacterial peritonitis in liver cirrhosis. Hepatology. 2010 Apr. 51(4):1327-33. [Medline].

3. Barretti P, Montelli AC, Batalha JE, Caramori JC, Cunha Mde L. The role of virulence factors in the outcome of staphylococcal peritonitis in CAPD patients. BMC Infect Dis. 2009 Dec 22. 9:212. [Medline]. [Full Text].

4. Bert F, Noussair L, Lambert-Zechovsky N, Valla D. Viridans group streptococci: an underestimated cause of spontaneous bacterial peritonitis in cirrhotic patients with ascites. Eur J Gastroenterol Hepatol. 2005 Sep. 17(9):929-33. [Medline].

5. Cholongitas E, Papatheodoridis GV, Lahanas A, Xanthaki A, Kontou-Kastellanou C, Archimandritis AJ. Increasing frequency of Gram-positive bacteria in spontaneous bacterial peritonitis. Liver Int. 2005 Feb. 25(1):57-61. [Medline].

6. Adler SN, Gasbarra DB. A Pocket Manual of Differential Diagnosis. Philadelphia, Pa: Lippincott Williams & Wilkins; 2005.

7. Nouri-Majalan N, Najafi I, Sanadgol H, et al. Description of an outbreak of acute sterile peritonitis in Iran. Perit Dial Int. 2010 Jan-Feb. 30(1):19-22. [Medline].

8. Evans LT, Kim WR, Poterucha JJ, Kamath PS. Spontaneous bacterial peritonitis in asymptomatic outpatients with cirrhotic ascites. Hepatology. 2003 Apr. 37(4):897-901. [Medline].

9. Cheruvattath R, Balan V. Infections in patients with end-stage liver disease. J Clin Gastroenterol. 2007 Apr. 41(4):403-11. [Medline].

Chapter 13

EMERGENCY LAPAROTOMY FOR TRAUMA

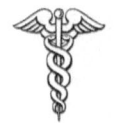

Ravi Kumar Garg

Abdominal trauma can be blunt or penetrating. depending on the nature of injuries patients are managed.

CAREFUL HISTORY OF

- Accident
- H/o alcohol or drug abuse
- Speed of vehicle

EXAMINATION OF

- level of consciousness for head injury
- examination of chest and ribs is very important
- examination of anterior, posterior and lateral walls of abdomen

- examination of lower chest, buttock and perineum for abrasions, laceration and penetrating wound

- examination of limbs

- Access for guarding and rigidity of abdominal wall

- Lower chest: intra thoracic abdomen for spleen rupture (Left side lower ribs)

- Liver – Rupture (Right side lower ribs)

- Diaphragm – for rupture and herniation of gut

- Stomach injury due to ruptured ribs, sternum injury, seatbelt injury

- Spleen rupture is most common in left lower chest trauma

- Abdomen injury - to small and large bowel

- Retroperitoneal: kidney, duodenum and pancreas, etc.

- Digital per rectal exam: is most important, look for presence of blood on the examining fingertip

- Vaginal examination in female patients

DIAGNOSTIC PERITONEAL LAVAGE (DPL)

Beneficial for occult injury in blunt trauma, not reliable for retroperitoneal haemorrhage

Contraindications:

H/o multiple abdominal surgeries previously

Is contraindicated in pregnancy, but an opening can be made above the uterus

In pelvic injury, also use supra umbilical approach

PROCEDURE

Through an infra umbilical catheter, 500 ml normal saline is infused in peritoneal cavity under gravity and drained back actively, and the fluid is examined (gross and microscopy).

Interpretations:

Laparotomy required: RBCs > 100,000/mm^3

WBC > 500/mm^3

Presence of bile, bacteria, faecal or vegetative matter

Negative DPL does not rule out retroperitoneal injuries

Laparotomy not required: if RBC < 50,000/mm^3

WBC < 100/mm^3

Open trauma/penetrating – always do laparotomy

Whether to do surgery or be conservative in blunt injuries to the abdomen depends upon:

Look – pale/pink

Pulse – fast, Thready

Shock

Distended abdomen

PLANNING OF EXPLORATION

Relevant pre-operative preparation of patient

Proper fluid

Antibiotic

Mostly midline incision

To convert to thoracoabdominal or not

Exploring abdomen in systematic way

Removing all clots/blood/fluids properly

DEFINING THE SITE OF INJURY

(for instance) Spleen rupture

Liver rupture

Mesentery tear

TACTICS OF EXPLORATION

Incision of abdomen heals from side to side and not from end to end

So, liberal midline incision

FIVE (P) TO STOP BLEEDING

Arrest bleeding by pressure/by packing.

Blood is scooped in cup shaped palm of hand. Insert the palm upwards and suck the blood in the concavity so created.

Eviscerate all small bowel loops upward and to the right over the right edge of a vertical incision of laparotomy, to inspect solid organ, and suck blood completely.

To find out perforation – eviscerate all small bowel upwards and to the right over the edge of a vertical laparotomy.

Pelvic blood/fluid is sucked out.

Inspect ascending, transverse and descending colon.

Open the lesser sac and examine posterior surface of stomach.

In extensive trauma to liver, segmental resection or segmentectomy is sometimes easier than attempts to stitch together shattered tissue.

In multiple and closely grouped perforation resection, anastomosis is better than individual repair.

DIAGNOSTIC LAPAROSCOPY

Can be done under LA or GA.

Diameter of scope as small as 4 mm to 10 mm,

Diagnosis by laparoscopy is better than peritoneal lavage in hemoperitoneum cases,

It reduces the incidence of negative laparotomy for patients with positive lavage findings.

For a patient with a previous laparotomy due to adhesion, USG and CT are best.

Neither DPL or laparoscopy can be done in these patients.

SPLENIC INJURY

Most common cause of hemoperitoneum - always ask if left shoulder tip referred pain is present.

Splenectomy should be avoided in children and young adults.

Enlarged spleen is more prone to rupture.

Clinical Presentation

- Rapid shock
- Hypovolemia - it can be accentuated by raising the head of bed.
- Thready, fast pulse
- Pale look
- Generalized pain and distended abdomen:
- Referred pain to left shoulder tip

Diagnosis

Paracentesis always +ve

X-ray chest - rupture of lower ribs - left

Elevated diaphragm Left

Enlarged splenic shadow

Medial displacement of gastric shadow

CT always diagnostic

Type of injury

Grade	Injury Description	Treatment Options
I	Capsular tear, < 1 cm parenchymal depth	Topical agents, argon beam coagulator
II	Capsular tear, 1–3 cm parenchymal depth that does not involve a trabecular vessel	Topical agents, argon beam coagulator
III	Laceration of >3 cm parenchymal depth involving trabecular vessels Ruptured subcapsular or parenchymal; intraparenchymal haematoma > 5 cm or expanding	Interrupted sutures, horizontal mattress sutures over a pedicle of omentum or Teflon pladgets, mesh splenorrhaphy
IV	Laceration involving segmental or hilar vessels producing major devascularization (>25% of spleen)	Partial splenectomy, mesh splenorrhaphy, splenectomy
V	Shattered spleen or hilar injury that devascularizes spleen	Splenectomy

In infants and children who are more prone to pneumococcal infection, H. infuenza and meningococcal infection after splenectomy, non-operative management may be tried and the spleen preserved

Operation

Midline laparotomy

Sub costal/thoracoabdominal incision for better exposure

First confirm the rupture of spleen by palpating with the right hand after sucking the blood

Left edge of laparotomy wound is retracted

Large pack is used to control transverse colon, splenic flex or/and small bowel

Blunt/sharp dissection of all adhesive

Deliver the spleen

Clamp the pedicle

Important: Care for the tail of pancreas. Make sure there is no injury

Mass ligature of pedicle should be avoided. A tube drain is always left in the splenic bed for 1–3 days after surgery

Always check the drain fluid for amylase in postoperative period, if injury to the tail of pancreas is suspected

Small Tears

Partial splenectomy - pack absorbable haemostatic material or omentum with sutures, enclose the spleen in synthetic absorbable material

Complications

- Serous collection in splenic bed
- Rx drainage by u/s or Ct guided needle
- Temporarily thrombocytosis
- Late infection OPSI oral chemotherapy
- Vaccination Pneumococcus, H. infuenzae, Meningococcal vaccine

LIVER INJURY

Next to spleen, liver injury is quiet common

Haemorrhage from liver is usually self-limiting, so conservative treatment is advised

Intervention is a advised when expending haematoma due to arterial bleed on serial CT examination

Diagram is by U/S CT

Paracentesis for hemoperitoneum

Grade		Injury Description
I	Haematoma	Subcapsular, 10% surface area
	Laceration	Capsular tear, 1 cm parenchymal depth
II	Haematoma	Subcapsular, 10–50% surface area; Intraparenchymal <10 cms in diameter

Grade		Injury Description
	Laceration	1–3 cms parenchymal depth
III	Haematoma	Subcapsular, >50% surface area or expanding; ruptured subcapsular or parenchymal haematoma
	Laceration	>3 cms parenchymal depth
IV	Laceration	Parenchymal disruption involving 25–75% of hepatic lobe Or 1–3 Couinaud`s segments within a lobe
V	Laceration	Parenchymal disruption involving >75% of hepatic lobe or More than 3 Couinaud`s segments within a single lobe
	Vascular	Juxtrahepatic venous injuries
VI	Vascular	Hepatic avulsion

NOMAT AS DESCRIBED

Surgical Intervention

Depending upon the type of injury midline/sub costal/ thoracoabdominal incision

Suck out blood

Pringle's manoeuvre for temporary stoppage of bleeding

Remove dead/devitalized liver tissue

Check for arterial spurt and do coagulation with cautery

Check for continuous venous ooze and do coagulation

Deep suture of liver tear – usually of not much use

If there is avulsion of hepatic veins from the inferior vena cava then massive uncontrolled bleeding occurs

Treatment of choice is judicious packing around the liver, so that the liver is sandwiched in the gauge packs all around

No packing inside the laceration

Balloon catheter can be inflated inside to tamponade the bleeding site. It acts as a drainage tube also for bile/blood.

Arterial bleeding : Difficult to control by packing

Treated by

- selecting angiography and embolization
- segmental resection
- selective hepatic artery ligation

Remove the pack on second laparotomy at 24–48 hours/may be extended up to 72 hours if bleeding persists

Complications

Late- parenchymal necrosis

Bile leaks

Haemobilia

Arterioportal fistula

Liver abscesses

Mesenteric Bleeding due to Injury

Mesenteric tear is the common cause of haemoperitoneum if spleen and liver are intact.

ALWAYS EXPLORE THE HAEMOPERTONEUM IN THE ABSENCE OF SOLID ORGAN INJURY

Management:

A large mesenteric haematoma requires gentle evacuation and ligation of the damaged vessel

Check for vitality of adjacent bowel loop of gut

Devascularized bowel must be resected

Retroperitoneal Haematoma

- **Zones of Retroperitoneum**
- Zone I
  - ➤ Diaphragmatic hiatus to sacral promontory
  - ➤ Contain major vessels
- Zone II
  - ➤ R & L Flanks
- Zone III
  - ➤ Pelvis

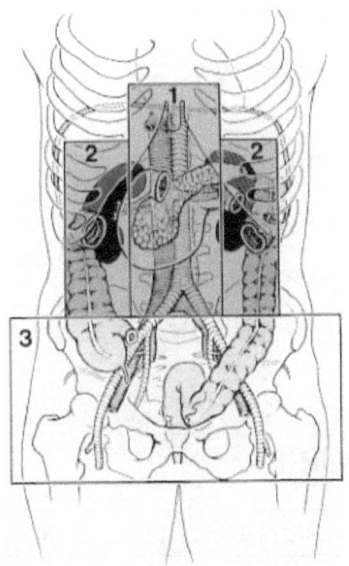

Photo Showing Various Zones

Treatment

- Always explore:
  - ➤ penetrating injuries
  - ➤ haematomas in Zone I
- Zone II – individualise
  - ➤ kidney, renovasculature
  - ➤ posterior colon
- Zone III
  - ➤ Pelvic retroperitoneal haematoma
  - ➤ Never explore

Selective vessel embolization

A non-expanding retroperitoneal haematoma can left untouched if

Distal flow is normal

> Not tear to a major vessel

> Not tear to pancreas

A expanding, pulsatile haematoma requires exploration

KIDNEY INJURIES

Grade	Injury Description	Treatment
I	Microscopic or gross haematuria, urologic studies normal Subcapsular haematoma, nonexpanding without parenchymal laceration	Observation
II	Nonexpanding perirenal haematoma confined to renal retroperitoneum Laceration of < 1 cm parenchymal depth of renal cortex without urinary extravasation	Observation Observation; perinephric drain
III	Laceration of >1 cm parenchymal depth of renal cortex without collecting system rupture or urinary extravasation	Debridement; ±closure; perinephric drain; omental patch

IV	Parenchymal laceration extending through the renal cortex, medulla, and collecting system with urinary extravasation Main renal artery or vein injury with contained hemorrhage	Repair collecting system; debridement; cortical closure; perinephric drain; omental patch repair; nephrectomy
V	Completely shattered kidney Avulsion of renal hilum that devascularizes kidney	Nephrectomy vs repair

Renal injuries result in retroperitoneal haematoma and haematuria

Conservative management in all renal injuries unless:

Expanding haematoma on CT

Decreasing haemoglobin

Haemodynamically unstable

Almost all renal injury heal by conservative management

If patient is unstable/open and do nephrectomy – partial or total

LAPAROTOMY AND DEFINITIVE REPAIR

1. Indications for laparotomy in a patient with blunt abdominal injury include signs of peritonitis, uncontrolled shock or haemorrhage,

clinical deterioration during observation, and hemoperitoneum findings after FAST or DPL examinations (see Workup).

2. When laparotomy is indicated, broad-spectrum antibiotics are given. A midline incision is usually preferred. When the abdomen is opened, haemorrhage control is accomplished by removing blood and clots, packing all four quadrants, and clamping vascular structures. Obvious hollow viscus injuries (HVIs) are sutured. After intra-abdominal injuries have been repaired and haemorrhage has been controlled by packing, a thorough exploration of the abdomen is then performed to evaluate the entire contents of the abdomen.

   After intraperitoneal injuries are controlled, the retroperitoneum and pelvis must be inspected.

3. Do not explore pelvic haematomas. Use external fixation of pelvic fractures to reduce or stop blood loss in this region. Explore large or expanding midline retroperitoneal haematomas, with the anticipation of damage to the large vascular structures, pancreas, or duodenum. Do not explore small or stable perinephric haematomas.

4. After the source of bleeding has been stopped, further stabilizing the patient with fluid resuscitation and appropriate warming is important. After such measures are complete, perform a thorough exploratory laparotomy with appropriate repair of all injured structures.

5. **It is safer to undergo laparotomy with negative findings than to delay treatment of an injury.** The true morbidity of a negative laparotomy may not be as high as previously believed. Exploratory laparotomy to establish a diagnosis does not result in increased morbidity in a 30-day period, compared with no laparotomy. **But avoid exploratory laparotomy if the CT is negative and the patient is haemodynamically stable.**

6. Patients who have gross enteric contamination of the peritoneal cavity are given appropriate antibiotics for 5–7 days.

7. If a pelvic haematoma is found and the patient continues to lose blood after external fixation of a pelvic fracture, arteriography with embolization can be used to stop the small percentage of arterial bleeding found in pelvic fractures.

8. In adults, splenic artery embolization has been shown to improve nonoperative splenic salvage rates. A retrospective review showed that this procedure may be useful in the adolescent population as well, particularly in patients with high-grade injuries or with evidence of splenic vascular injury, although this is not the standard of care. [47]

9. The best results were attained if the reoperation took place within 24 hours of the initial surgery A multicenter study found that delays in returning to the operating room after damage control laparotomy are associated with the failure to achieve primary fascial closure.

10. Specific physical examination findings that call for timely surgical evaluation are as follows:

- History of blunt abdominal trauma, shock, or abnormal vital signs (e.g., tachycardia, hypotension)

- Evidence of shock without obvious external blood loss

- Evidence of peritonitis (e.g., marked tenderness, involuntary guarding, percussion tenderness)

- Findings consistent with potential intra-abdominal injury (e.g., lap belt signs, lower rib fractures, lumbar spine fractures)

- Altered levels of consciousness or sensation, whether due to drugs, alcohol, or head/spinal injury

- Patients who require other prolonged operative intervention (e.g., orthopaedic procedures)

Specific findings on diagnostic studies that call for timely surgical evaluation include evidence of free fluid or solid organ injury on sonograms or CT scans.

Although a trend toward nonoperative management of hepatic, splenic, and renal injuries in patients who are haemodynamically normal has occurred, a trained trauma surgeon must oversee this care.

11. Other specific findings that indicate timely trauma surgeon involvement are as follows:

- Positive findings on DPL

- Evidence of extravasated contrast or extraluminal air on an upper gastrointestinal series (e.g., duodenal rupture), plain abdominal radiography, or cystography

- Serious pelvic fractures

- Evidence of bladder rupture on contrast cystogram or gross haematuria

- Elevated findings on liver function studies

12. Lengthy diagnostic workup is counterproductive once it is recognized that a patient cannot be managed at the initial facility. Shift the patients as early as possible. Physician-to-physician consultation must occur before transport to ensure that the receiving facility has the resources necessary to care for the patient.

13. Before discharge, provide patients with detailed instructions that describe signs of undiagnosed injury. Increased abdominal pain or distention, nausea or vomiting, weakness, lightheadedness or fainting, or new bleeding in urine or feces mandates immediate return and further evaluation. Ensure that close follow-up care and repeat examinations are available for all patients.

NONOPERATIVE MANAGEMENT OF ABDOMINAL TRAUMA (NOMAT)

- Patient should be haemodynamically stable

- Charting of pulse, blood pressure, respiration rate, abdominal girth

- Non expending haematoma on CT

- RT Aspiration, nil per oral

- Serial haemoglobin check up

- Prophylactic broad spectrum antibiotics

- Catheterize patient to measure output

- Serial U/S or CT examination

- Blood should be transfused

REFERENCES

1. Chereau N, Wagner M, Tresallet C, Lucidarme O, Raux M, Menegaux F. CT scan and Diagnostic Peritoneal Lavage: towards a better diagnosis in the area of nonoperative management of blunt abdominal trauma. Injury. 2016 Sep;47 (9):2006-11. doi: 10.1016/j.injury. 2016.04.034.

2. Kohler JE, Chokshi NK. Management of Abdominal Solid Organ Injury After Blunt Trauma. Pediatr Ann. 2016 Jul 1;45(7):e241-6. doi: 10.3928/00904481-20160518-01.

3. Girard E, Abba J, Cristiano N, Siebert M, Barbois S, Létoublon C etal. Management of splenic and pancreatic trauma. J Visc Surg. 2016 Aug;153 (4 Suppl):45-60. doi: 10.1016/j.jviscsurg.2016.04.005.

4. Notrica DM, Linnaus ME. Nonoperative Management of Blunt Solid Organ Injury in Paediatric Surgery. Surg Clin North Am. 2017 Feb;97(1):1-20. doi: 10.1016/j.suc.2016.08.001. Review.

Chapter 14

PEARLS ABOUT ABDOMINAL WOUND CLOSURE

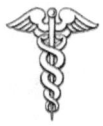

Gaurav Thami

"There are few things more embarrassing to a surgeon than the sight of his recently operated patient, his abdomen gaping, and the gut spilling out all around..."

Moshe Schein

Healing of abdominal incisions is similar to the healing of other wounds. The inflammatory phase lasts for approximately four days, followed by the proliferative phase for three weeks. The maturation phase continues for up to a year. Healing of the abdominal wall fascia by end of two weeks is 20%; by the end of four weeks, is nearly 50%; at eight weeks is about 60–80%; and after 52 weeks, up to 90% of the healing takes place.

After 2–4 weeks, the healing fascia begins to have the strength to be self-supporting but is still vulnerable to wound dehiscence. Thus, the abdominal wall attains 52–59% of its original strength in 42 days, 70–80% in 120 days, and 73–93% by 140 days. Maximum strength finally achieved is 93% of the original strength. Thus, healing fascia requires at least 14 to 28 days before becoming self-supportive. This time is also known as the "critical healing period". Disruptions in any of the phases of wound healing can lead to wound complications or can result in severely reduced strength of healing fascia. These disruptions can be due to localized infections or can be attributed to delayed healing due to patient factors such as diabetes or smoking. The wound is at its weakest on postoperative day 3. Postoperatively, abdominal fascia will never completely regain its original strength. [1,2]

Despite many advances in surgical techniques, equipment, and supplies, complications after abdominal wall closure remain a persistent problem. The ideal abdominal closure should be efficient, provide strength, and serve as a barrier to infection. It should have low rates of fascial dehiscence, infection, hernia formation, suture sinus formation, and incisional pain. Decreasing local wound complications and incisional hernia formation after abdominal wound closure remains a persistent challenge.

A recent study evaluating surgery residents found that only 10% of residents knew the correct suture-to-wound-length ratio, and only 40% were familiar with literature on the proper technique of abdominal closure. Thus, if incisional hernia rates are to be decreased, education regarding current best practices of abdominal closure need to be addressed.

SURGICAL ANATOMY OF THE ABDOMINAL WALL

The abdominal wall is a musculoaponeurotic structure through which surgeons can often feel diseased organs that lie within the abdominal cavity. An intact abdominal wall is essential for the support of the abdominal contents. A defect or malfunction of the wall can allow the abdominal contents to bulge forward and form an incisional hernia. The abdominal wall also provides the surgeon with a site for access to deep-lying diseased structures. The anatomic principle governs the incisions used for laparotomy. During respiration, coughing, sneezing, a temporary rise in intra-abdominal pressure occurs, which, following surgery, can result in any of the above complications, if due attention is not paid to prevent them.

Across the abdominal wall, stretch the linea transverse, tendinous intersections which in more muscular persons, produce palpable transverse depressions. These depressions are accentuated in active rectus contractions or in reflex muscle spasms associated with irritation of the peritoneum. At the lateral margin of each rectus muscle is a depression, linea semilunaris, directed towards the symphysis, the pubic tubercle is palpable at the medial attachments of the inguinal ligaments, located about two fingers breadth above suspensory ligament of penis and about 2.5 cm lateral to midline.

The abdominal wall is composed of nine layers:

1. Skin

2. Subcutaneous fatty layer

3. Scarpa's superficial fascia

4. External oblique muscle

5. Internal oblique muscle

6. Transversus abdominis muscle

7. Transversalis fascia (endo abdominal fascia)

8. Extra peritoneal adipose and loose areolar tissue

9. Peritoneum

Abdominal Incisions and Closure

A wisely chosen incision, correct methods of making and closing such wounds are factors of great importance. A badly placed incision cutting the motor nerves supplying abdominal musculature, clumsy methods of suturing, ill-judged selection of suture materials and bad technique of closure may all result in serious complications like haematoma formation, infection, stitch abscess, ugly scar formation, incisional hernia or, worst of all, the complete disruption of wound. The surgeons aim is to employ the type of incision depending on the surgery being performed. However, the three essentials of an incision are that it should have accessibility, extensibility and security.

General Principles

- The incision must give ready and direct access to the anatomy to be investigated. It must also provide adequate room for the procedure to be performed.

- The incision should be extensible, if need arises, in a direction that will allow for any probable enlargement of the scope of operation. However, it should interfere as little as possible with the function of abdominal wall in future.

- Security is the most important principle governing any abdominal surgery, hence closure of the abdominal wound must be reliable. Ideally it should leave the abdominal wall as strong after the operation as before.

- Drains, when used, are inserted through a stab wound away from the incision, and a colostomy or ileostomy when performed, is always fashioned through a separate incision.

- Wide bites must be taken at a minimum 1 cm from the wound edge and placed at an interval of 1 cm or less.

- The suture length should measure at least four times the wound length to ensure an adequate reserve of suture length in the wound, when the suture is placed on tensions as may occur during abdominal distension

- Strict aseptic precautions should be taken to prevent contamination of the wound and subsequent infection

Closure technique involves a choice of continuous versus interrupted sutures, the size of fascial bites, distance between consecutive sutures (stitch interval) and the length and size of the suture used. The mechanical characteristics of different suture techniques have a direct influence on wound strength. Simple interrupted suture (SIS) is the traditionally used technique for closure of laparotomy wounds. The disadvantages of SIS are - the greater amount of suture material used, and overall time involved in tying and cutting numerous knots. Suture material contained in SIS is mostly in the form of knots which makes that part of the tissue subject to foreign body reaction and wound infection.

Interrupted double loop closure (IDLC) and simple continuous suture (SCS) techniques are used often. The IDLC improves wound strength by creating tension on the inner loops of the suture, which keeps the incision edges in close approximation. Wounds closed by IDLC can tolerate higher intra-abdominal pressure than those closed using the SCS technique.

The advantages of a continuous suture are speed, an equal distribution of tension, less foreign material in the wound, and less wound trauma.

Various types of suture techniques used in clinical practice are:

- Simple interrupted suture (SIS)

- Simple continuous suture (SCS)

- Interrupted double loop closure (IDLC)

- Continuous double loop closure (CDLC)

The following principles should be used while using different suture techniques:

- Wound closure should be started from the cranial end of the incision and suture intervals should be 1 cm for all techniques.

- Suture bites should be taken 5 mm from the incision edge. In IDLC and CDLC, far bites should be placed at 5 mm, and near bites at 2.5 mm from the edge of the incision.

- All sutures should pass through all musculoaponeurotic layers and peritoneum. Interrupted sutures should be tied with a 2x1x1 square knot.

- Continuous sutures are anchored at the cranial pole of the wound with a 2x1x1x1 square knot and at the caudal pole of the wound with a 2×1×1×1×1 square knot.

- The sutures should be tied with just enough tension to loosely approximate the rectus sheath.

- All knots should be positioned away from the incisional region in order not to interfere with the regenerative process.

- The suture length required to close the wounds is determined by suture length along the wound, in the knots and in the knot ends (ears).

CLOSURE OF MIDLINE INCISION

Mass Closure

The mass closure technique of midline incision consists of suturing of the cut edges of the peritoneum and linea alba together. Care is taken to take wide bites of the cut edges, at least 1 cm from the edge of the incision and a handheld 5/8 cutting needle is used and continuous locking sutures taken, using polypropylene no. 1. The skin is sutured with fine interrupted nylon; deep tension sutures are not used.

Layered Closure

In this technique the peritoneum is closed by continuous interlocking sutures. The linea alba is closed similarly with polypropylene no. 1 by continuous interlocking sutures.

CLOSURE OF PARAMEDIAN INCISIONS

Mass Closure

In this technique the peritoneum, endo abdominal fascia, posterior layer of rectus sheath, rectus abdominus and anterior layer of rectus sheath are all sutured as a single layer. The bites are taken at least 1 cm from the edge of the incision and a hand held 5/8 cutting needle is used. Continuous locking sutures are employed using polypropylene no. 1.

Layered Closure

In this technique, the peritoneum and the posterior layer of rectus sheath are closed with continuous interlocking sutures. The anterior layer of rectus sheath is closed by continuous interlocking.

4. TEMPORARY ABDOMINAL CLOSURE TECHNIQUES

Skin-Only Closure Techniques. The temporary skin-only closure techniques use the skin to provide some abdominal wall stability with containment of abdominal viscera. These techniques use a series of towel clips or a rapid monofilament running suture. The towel clip closure is perhaps the most rapid of the temporary closure techniques. The towel clips are applied to the skin, approximately 1 cm apart. Either towel clips or suture closure of the skin is swift, inexpensive, and easily available. The abdominal contents are maintained below the level of the fascia, which minimizes heat and fluid loss. However, as the bursting pressure of the skin is low, both techniques have increased risks of evisceration, injury and loss of skin, infection, and recurrent ACS.

Bogota Bag. When skin-only closure is impossible, as is often the case, a temporary plastic Bogota bag, sutured to the skin, provides an excellent solution for containment. After the initial operation, a pre-sterilized, soft 3-L IV bag is cut to an oval shape and stapled with a standard skin stapling device or sutured with monofilament suture to the skin edges of the wound. Sterile, antibiotic-soaked towels are placed over the silo, which is then covered with an iodine-impregnated adhesive plastic drape. The wound is inspected and the dressing is changed every 24 hours.

Other alternatives include bowel bag, Steri-Drape, or Silastic cloth. These materials hold sutures or staples well, help to retain body heat, minimize fluid loss, are quick and easy to apply, and are non-irritating to the underlying viscera. A silo closure may decrease respiratory and renal compromise associated with a decrease in intra-abdominal pressure. The Bogota bag closure is much less expensive than any other techniques which are currently available. The technique may be particularly useful for surgeons who encounter severe abdominal trauma in small rural hospitals, because life-saving interventions, such as control of bleeding, need to be performed immediately and rapidly before the patients are transferred to a major hospital for definitive treatment. However, Bogota bags do not prevent abdominal wall retraction, and they do not allow effective removal of abdominal fluids.

Mesh. Permanent synthetic prostheses, when sutured to the fascial edges, can be used to protect abdominal wall tissues from the damages which result from repetitive surgical procedures through the incision, prevent lateral retraction of the fascia, and facilitate reoperation. However, wrinkling secondary to wound contracture, infection, hernia, mesh extrusion, and enterocutaneous fistula are some of the complications that may ensue.

Several permanent synthetic repair materials are available, including the broad classes of macroporous, microporous, and composite materials. Although meshes improved the primary closure rates which ranged from 33 to 89%, macroporous repair materials such as polypropylene were associated with a high incidence of 6.6% to 14.7% of fistulas when placed in contact with the bowel. Nonadherent materials should be placed between the intra-abdominal contents and fascia to prevent formation of fistulas and to facilitate future manipulation of the wound. Microporous repair materials such as polytetrafluoroethylene (ePTFE) which resists adherence to tissues may be used over the bowel.

The main disadvantage of microporous repair materials is the increased risk of infection. Absorbable meshes include polyglactin 910 (Vicryl; Ethicon, Somerville, NJ) and polyglycolic acid]. The advantages of an absorbable mesh are as follows: it is resistant to infection, pliable, and easier to work with than the currently available permanent meshes. The mesh does not unravel when cut and can be opened repeatedly to provide less traumatic access to the abdominal cavity for repeated drainage procedures.. However, the use of absorbable meshes has resulted in fistula formation rates which ranged from 5% to 11% and intra-abdominal abscesses.

Gore Bio-A mesh has a web of biocompatible synthetic polymers which are gradually absorbed in six months. The use of Gore Bio-A is safe, feasible, and cost-effective, even within a contaminated field. Unlike the permanent meshes, it facilitates ingrowth of granulation tissues causing the covering to adhere to the wound.

Wittmann Patch. The Wittmann Patch, consists of two detachable components—a loop sheet and a closure sheet. Firm pressure causes penetration of the free ends of the "mushrooms" of the closure sheet through the loop sheet, creating a stable configuration between them. The burr can be opened by peeling, but it withstands shearing forces across the laparotomy. Typically, the patch is sequentially tightened every 24–48 hours until the fascia is approximately 2–4 cm apart. Then this temporary closure is removed at the final operation and some form of definitive closure is used to close the fascia primarily.

Many methods have been advocated to maintain abdominal integrity and to facilitate fascial approximation, including the use of zippers, slide fasteners, and a Velcro analogue. The mesh, zippers, or Wittmann Patch permits rapid and safe re-entry into the abdomen on re-exploration, and if additional laparotomy is necessary in the future, permits a rapid closure. The opening and closure of the Wittmann Patch takes only seconds. Other advantages of the Wittmann Patch technique include a gradual approximation of fascia, ease of re-exploration, and prevention of loss of abdominal domain. The Wittmann Patch technique is more costly and requires suturing to the abdominal fascia, which may increase the risk of fascial trauma and necrosis, and future incisional hernias may develop. Finally, this technique does not effectively evacuate peritoneal fluid, and abdominal wound drainage may become an issue.

Vacuum-Assisted Closure. Negative pressure therapy (NPT) has been shown to increase local blood perfusion and nutrient delivery to the wound, accelerate growth of granulation tissues, and decrease wound bacterial concentrations. It also reduces bowel oedema and the application of mechanical stress to the wound and accelerates cellular proliferation and angiogenesis. The negative pressure therapy, by the principle of reverse tissue expansion in the wound, brings together the wound edges.

Vacuum-assisted closure consists of four component layers: The first layer is a perforated polyethylene sheet that is placed beneath the peritoneum of the abdominal wall. This material provides some protection to the viscera, and the non-adherent nature of the polyethylene prevents adhesion of the viscera to itself and to the under surface of the abdominal. The second layer consists of suction drains and compressible material, either sterile surgical towels or polyurethane foam. When negative pressure is applied to the dressing, these materials become semirigid, thus providing additional protection and preventing fascial retraction by creating a constant medial tension on the fascia without suture. The third layer consists of silicone drains placed above the towels/ sponges and serve as a negative pressure source and a means of controlling egress of intra-abdominal fluid. The drains are connected to a negative pressure source of 100 to 150 mm Hg. The fourth layer is an adhesive sheet which serves to cover the skin surrounding the wound and complete the vacuum seal. The dressing is maintained intact under suction until re-exploration. The two most commonly used negative-pressure dressings systems are the V.A.C. Abdominal Dressing System and AB Thera System from KCI.

VACUUM-ASSISTED WOUND CLOSURE AND MESH-MEDIATED FASCIAL TRACTION

This is a new technique which combines the vacuum pack technique with continuous medial fascial traction through a Wittmann patch sutured to the edges of the fascia, thus leading to a higher incidence of fascia-to-fascia abdominal wall closure. The VAWCM technique can be successfully used in septic patients, even when the wound is complex and/or contaminated.

FASCIAL BRIDGE TECHNIQUES FOR PRIMARY FASCIAL CLOSURE

Closure of the fascia should be performed without undue tension because excessive tension on fascial closure can result in increased IAP, ventral hernia, or fascial dehiscence. As described above, through the appropriate use of the TAC techniques, patients with open abdomen can undergo multiple reoperations with progressive and final closure of the fascial defect. However, for patients who have ongoing intra-abdominal infection, visceral oedema, loss of abdominal domain or fascia, or complicated wound problems; delayed abdominal fascial closure (DAFC) may not be possible. Under such conditions, the limited available surgical options include performing an acute abdominal wall reconstruction using the component separation technique; bridge repair of fascial defect using synthetic/ prosthetic mesh or biologic mesh; or a planned ventral hernia.

COMPONENT SEPARATION

Reconstruction of the midline defect with an innervated advancement of muscle and fascia. The technique consists of the following:

1. anterior abdominal wall skin flaps are developed and dissected from the anterior superior iliac spines to the chest wall

2. the aponeurosis of the external oblique muscle is divided lateral to the semilunar line at the level of the xiphoid

3. the external oblique is feed, which will allow the rectus myofascial component to be mobilized medially

4. the midline is sutured together. This technique facilitates release of the lateral oblique muscles and is helpful in closing persistent fascial defects.

Bilateral advancement yields enough mobility to close defects of 10 cm in the epigastrium, 20 cm at the umbilicus, and 6 cm at the suprapubic level. However, its use for acute definitive closure in the setting of open abdomen has not been well studied. In severe intra-abdominal sepsis, visceral and abdominal wall oedema, and ongoing systemic sepsis, component separation is not advisable.

FASCIAL BRIDGE USING PROSTHETIC MESH

Polypropylene mesh is highly effective in the early restoration of abdominal wall continuity.

Tension free repair of large ventral hernias with prosthetic mesh is associated with hernia recurrence rates which ranged from 2% to 18%, and complication rates which range from 10% to 17%. The association of prosthetic mesh with bacterial colonization is well known, which has been reported to be up to 6.8% even in the absence of contamination.

Biologic Mesh. Prosthetic mesh allows for a tension free repair of the fascial defect. Unfortunately, it is associated with a completely different set of problems. In addition, it does not bring any of the basic wound healing units (e.g., glycosaminoglycans, fibronectin) into the wound field. The mesh becomes only minimally integrated in the final wound and it is never truly an integrated implant. Several approaches have been developed in an attempt to address these problems. Local flaps, pedicle or free flaps, have been utilized to provide additional soft tissue coverage and the necessary ingredients for wound healing. However, it cannot be applied universally, even if successful in some patients. The fascial defect may be too large for these tissue flaps to cover. Autologous tissue is neither always available nor it is free of donor morbidity. Postoperative complications and reherniation still are troublesome problems with rates ranging from 0% to 43% and 8% to 32%, respectively. Therefore, an ideal prosthesis is one that augments the body's natural efforts to heal, provides structural support, allows for ingrowth, and is eventually replaced or fully integrated.

Many of these characteristics are found in acellular dermal matrix (ADM). ADM is a biologic material derived from a donor source—which in most cases is human cadaveric, porcine, or bovine in origin. ADM has a special ability to integrate into the native tissue, which helps in wound strength and offers a more biocompatible solution. In addition, in the absence of a permanent prosthetic mesh at the repair site, ADM also shows excellent mechanical properties, such as tensile strength, plasticity and flexibility. One of the most prominent concerns with ADM is that it stretches over time, leading to abdominal wall laxity and recurrent hernia, ranging widely from 0% to 80%.

Eight Pearls to decrease local wound complications and hernia formation after laparotomy wound closure:

1. Fascial closure with a size 1 or 2, slowly absorbable monofilament suture should be used.

2. Wound should be closed in one layer, in a continuous manner, with self-locking anchor knots.

3. The suture length-to-wound-length ratio should be greater than 4:1. Closure should be accomplished with small fascial bites (5–8 mm). Fascial bites should be 1 cm from the fascial edges and have half cm advances.

4. Excessive tension should be avoided. Just approximate the wound.

5. Obtaining the appropriate ratio and smaller fascial bites can more easily be done if a smaller suture and needle are used.

6. The use of prophylactic mesh in certain high-risk patient populations is a reasonable consideration. [3]

7. The age-old practice of using tension sutures when dehiscence is anticipated should not be encouraged, and, in fact, should not be used. There is a risk of producing "bow string" damage to the bowel coming in contact with these tight sutures, and, also, the associated tension may actually hurt the cause.

8. Every abdomen should not be closed. In the event of poor sepsis scores/APACHE scores, with the possibility of abdominal compartment syndrome, avoid closure of the abdomen as it will open up on its own. It can cause an irreversible physiological damage. Such abdomens are better managed as open abdomens, or laparostomies, with or without any zippers.

In spite of the best wound closure technique, there can be wound dehiscence. Due to various patient risk factors.

PATIENT RISK FACTORS

Demographic risk factors for dehiscence and incisional hernia are similar. These risks include obesity, advanced age, male sex, smoking, diabetes mellitus, malnutrition, malignancy, and steroid use.[4] These factors may contribute to delayed wound healing and decreased collagen synthesis. The effect of interventions focused on modifiable risk factors such as smoking and obesity remain a clinical challenge.

Steroid or immunosuppressive therapy can have deleterious effects on wound healing, with patients undergoing liver transplantation reported to have incisional hernia rates of up to 23%.[5]

Relaparotomy is another strong risk factor for postoperative incisional hernia formation. This may be due to resuturing of relatively nonvascular scar tissue leading to insufficient healing.

Postoperative wound infections are one of the most well-documented risk factors for early dehiscence and subsequent hernia formation. The proliferation of bacteria leads to decreased collagen synthesis and weakening of the fascial closure.[6] Postoperative abdominal distention and respiratory failure are also major risk factors for dehiscence and hernia formation. Distention increases tension along the suture line, causing higher risk of suture breaking, knot slipping, and suture cutting through the fascia and soft tissue. Loosening of the suture and separation of the fascial edges can lead to incisional hernia formation.

Take Home Message

1. No tension

2. Single Layer Closure

   • incorporating fascia and no muscle

3. Jenkins' Rule of 4

   • 2cm by 2cm

4. Continuous vs Interrupted

   If high risk of wound infection then use interrupted

REFERENCES

1. Hardy MA. The biology of scar formation. *Phys Ther*. 1989;69:1014–1024.

2. Chintamani Editorial: Ten Commandments of Safe and Optimum Abdominal Wall Closure. Indian Journal of Surgery (April 2018) 80(2):105–108 https://doi.org/10.1007/s12262-018-1776-6

3. Caro-Tarrago A, Olona Casas C, Jimenez Salido A, et al. Prevention of incisional hernia in midline laparotomy with an onlay mesh: a randomized clinical trial. *World J Surg*. 2014;38(9):2223–2230.

4. Ashcroft GS, Horan MA, Ferguson MW. Aging is associated with reduced deposition of specific extracellular matrix components, an upregulation

of angiogenesis, and an altered inflammatory response in a murine incisional wound healing model. *J Invest Dermatol.* 1997;108:430–437

5. Kahn J, Muller H, Iberer F, et al. Incisional hernia following liver transplantation: incidence and predisposing factors. *Clin Transplant.* 2007;21:423–426.

6. Graham DJ, Stevenson JT, McHenry CR. The association of intra-abdominal infection and abdominal wound dehiscence. *Am Surg.* 1998;64:660–665.

Chapter 15

ABDOMINAL COMPARTMENT SYNDROME

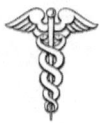

Dr Yamani

LEARNING OBJECTIVE

To understand

- What is Abdominal Compartment Syndrome (ACS) and Intra-Abdominal Hypertension (IAH)

- Its etiology, diagnosis and management

INTRODUCTION

The abdominal compartment syndrome (ACS) is defined as increasing abdominal organ dysfunction or failure due to high intra-abdominal pressure. It is a major cause of high morbidity and mortality in critically ill patients - therefore, early diagnosis and management is essential as it is reversible. High intra-abdominal pressure leads to low abdominal perfusion pressure (APP), poor blood flow and tissue ischemia, which contributes to multiple organ failure.

In healthy individuals, normal IAP is <5–7 mm Hg.[1] In case of morbid obesity and pregnancy it may rise to 10-15 mm Hg without any complication. The ACS is defined as the presence of Urinary Bladder Pressure (UBP) of > 20 mm Hg with cardiovascular (DO_2I < 600 ml O2/min/m2), pulmonary (peak airway pressure > 45 cmH2O), and/or renal dysfunction i.e. urinary output (UOP) < 0.5 ml/kg/hr. The ACS developed within 27 ± 4 hours with a UBP of 27 ± 2.3 mm Hg.

Abdominal perfusion pressure (APP) = Mean arterial pressure (MAP) – Intra-abdominal pressure (IAP). Target APP should be 60 mm of Hg for good survival rate.

Renal filtration gradient = Mean arterial pressure – 2* intra-abdominal pressure.

According to the level of IAP, IAH (Intra-Abdominal Hypertension) is graded as follows: [2]

Grade I: IAP 12–15 mm Hg – may be asymptomatic depending on the intra-arterial blood pressure and abdominal wall compliance

Grade II: IAP 16–20 mm Hg

Grade III: IAP 21–25 mm Hg

Grade IV: IAP >25 mm Hg - individual is prone to ACS

Intraabdominal hypertension and abdominal compartment syndrome

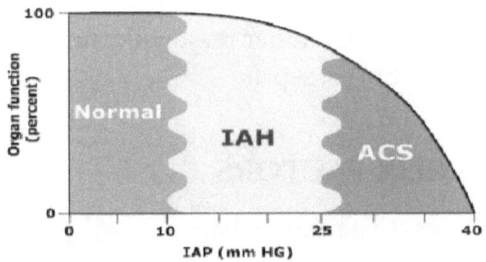

Intraabdominal hypertension (IAH) is defined as a sustained intraabdominal pressure >12 mmHg. Abdominal compartment syndrome (ACS) is defined as a sustained intraabdominal pressure>20 mmHg that is associated with new organ dysfunction. *Based on information from: Abdominal perfusion pressure.* AdominalCompartmentSyndrome.org

IAH can be:

Hyper acute –lasts for a few seconds as during coughing or sneezing.

Acute – develops over hours as during abdominal trauma.

Subacute – seen in medical conditions.

Chronic – in morbid obesity or pregnancy. These individuals are more prone to ACS if there is acute chronically raised intra-abdominal pressure (IAP). Decrease in abdominal wall compliance helps in prevention of ACS till threshold is reached.

Recently, it has been found that even lower levels of raised IAP can cause adverse effects and become evident prior to the development of severe ACS. It has isolated effects on gut perfusion and thus oxygenation.

ACS can be:

Primary – due to intra-abdominoperineal pathology like abdominal trauma, peritonitis etc.

Secondary – due to any other reason like fluid correction with crystalloid, burns, sepsis.

VARIOUS RISK FACTORS

- Postoperative haemorrhage
- Oedema after extensive dissection
- Reduction of diaphragmatic hernia
- Tight fascial closure of abdomen
- Increased intra-abdominal abdominal pressure during laparoscopy
- Paralytic ileus
- Intra-abdominal abscesses
- Post traumatic
- Poly-transfusion
- Excessive fluid resuscitation
- Acute pancreatitis
- Space occupying mass abdomen
- Gastric dilatation
- Peritoneal dialysis

AETIOLOGY

There are many causes of acutely elevated IAP pressure. The ACS develops with acute and rapid (i.e., in hours) elevation in IAP. Chronic increase in intra-abdominal volume, as in morbidly obese patients, lead to a slower increase in IAP. In these cases the abdominal wall accommodates and becomes more compliant with time, the phenomenon of 'stress-relaxation'. With this gradual increase, the various organ systems are able to compensate for the changes in IAP. Consequently, the acute deterioration seen with ACS does not occur in these patients. However, this does not mean that elevated IAP in these individuals is benign.

Acute:	
Retroperitoneal Origin	Pancreatitis, pelvic or retroperitoneal bleeding, contained abdominal aortic aneurysm rupture, aortic surgery, abscess, visceral oedema
Intra-peritoneal Origin	Intraperitoneal bleeding, free abdominal aortic aneurysm rupture, acute gastric dilatation, bowel obstruction, ileus, mesenteric venous obstruction, pneumoperitoneum, abdominal packing, abscess, visceral oedema
Abdominal Wall	Burn eschar, repair of gastroschisis or omphalocele, reduction of large hernias, military anti-shock garments, laparotomy closure under extreme tension
Chronic:	Central obesity, ascites, large abdominal tumours, chronic ambulatory peritoneal dialysis, pregnancy

CLINICAL FEATURES

Abdominal compartment syndrome can be diagnosed when there is evidence of organ dysfunction in combination with increased IAP.

In primary ACS, diagnosis may be missed as patient is severely ill.

Secondary ACS may be diagnosed in patients with fluid overload, burns and sepsis, by observing the following features:

- Difficulty in breathing
- Difficult ventilation
- Rising pulmonary artery pressure (PAP)
- Hypercapnia
- Hypoxia
- Oliguria (later)
- Reduced cardiac output despite high filling pressure
- Abdomen distended and tense
- Neurological deterioration
- Raised CVP, PCWP and PAP and acidosis
- Anuria, ventricular failure, cardiac decompensation
- Death

INVESTIGATIONS

- Measurement of intra-abdominal pressure

THROUGH URINARY BLADDER PRESSURE – GOLD STANDARD

This technique was first described by Kron, where pressure can be measured by placing a three-way Foley catheter in the urinary bladder. The bladder is drained and then filled with 50 to 100 ml of sterile saline. The Foley catheter is used with an adapter for the connection. Using pubic symphysis as the zero-reference point, the tubing is attached to a water manometer or pressure transducer. This technique has been validated in animal studies showing a high degree of correlation with directly measured IAP (r = +0.85–0.98, p < 0.001) over a wide range of IAP up to 70 mm Hg. It is an easy method to use to carry out tests as well, as it provides a high degree of correlation over wide ranges of IAP. However, a small neurogenic bladder or intraperitoneal adhesions may make UBP unreliable at estimating IAP. This test is fall positive in chronic increases in IAP, secondary to central obesity, pregnancy or ascites. Bladder pressure measurements are not possible in patients with bladder trauma, neurogenic bladders, outflow obstruction and tense pelvic haematomas.

1. A nasogastric IAP monitor has been developed as well.[3] Measurement through the stomach has some advantages; it avoids problems associated with creating a hydrostatic fluid column in the bladder and is easier for continuous measurement. Due to progressive acute rises in IAP, ACS develops and affects intra-abdominal organs. The intestine is the most sensitive to IAH and develops evidence of end-organ damage, prior to the development of the classic renal, pulmonary, and cardiovascular signs.

2. Other investigations – Gastric mucosal pH, near-infrared spectroscopy to measure muscle and tissue oxygenation

Management- [2]

- Treatment involves decompression of the abdomen – otherwise due to reduced oxygen delivery, multiple organ failure occurs which leads to death. ACS is mostly encountered due to massive volume resuscitation in multiple trauma with massive blood loss and/or in prolonged surgeries. The knowledge of ACS is also essential to understanding the limitations of laparoscopy when there is high abdominal pressure.

- Monitoring of IAP: If a patient is resuscitated with 6 litres of fluid in six hours, measurement of IAP is a must. Other important parameters are BP, urine output and APP.

- Optimization of systemic perfusion.

- Specific medical management to reduce IAP and

- Swift surgical decompression for refractory IAH.

- Serial IAP measurements are necessary to guide resuscitation of patients with IAH/ACS.

- Fluid resuscitation volume should be continuously monitored to avoid over-resuscitation in patients at risk for IAH/ACS.

- Hypertonic crystalloid and colloid-based resuscitation are used in patients with IAH to decrease the progression to secondary ACS.

- Diuretic therapy, in combination with colloid, may be considered to mobilize third-space oedema, following initial resuscitation, once the patient is haemodynamically stable.

- Percutaneous catheter decompression should be considered in patients with intraperitoneal fluid, abscess, or blood, who demonstrate symptomatic IAH or ACS. Percutaneous catheter insertion under ultrasound guidance allows ongoing drainage of intraperitoneal fluid and may help avoid the need for open abdominal decompression in selected patients with secondary ACS.

- Escharotomy in severe burns.

- Surgical decompression should be performed in patients with ACS that is refractory to other treatment options (Grade 1B). Various surgical options are-

  ➤ Muscle relaxing incision (like fasciotomy).

  ➤ Avoid primary closure of abdomen – closure can be done by skin flaps only creating iatrogenic ventral hernia, closure by composite mesh or bioprosthesis or by tissue expander, myocutaneous flaps etc.

Take Home Message

To summarize, Abdominal Compartment Syndrome (ACS) is a life-threatening emergency that manifests due to severe intra-abdominal hypertension (IAH)which is reversible if diagnosed and managed early.

Recommendations for further reading :

Bailey and Love's - Short Practice of Surgery

Sabiston's - Textbook of Surgery

REFERENCES

1. Sugrue M. Abdominal compartment syndrome. Curr Opin Crit Care. 2005; 11:333–8. [PubMed] [Google Scholar]

2. Theodossis S Papavramidis, Athanasios D Marinis,[1] Ioannis Pliakos, Isaak Kesisoglou, and Nicki Papavramidou2 Abdominal compartment syndrome – Intra-abdominal hypertension: Defining, diagnosing, and managing. J Emerg Trauma Shock. 2011 Apr-Jun; 4(2): 279–291.doi: 10.4103/0974-2700.82224

3. Reed SF, Britt RC, Collins J, Weireter L, Cole F, Britt LD. Aggressive surveillance and early catheter-directed therapy in the management of intra-abdominal hypertension. J Trauma. 2006; 61:1359–65. [PubMed] [Google Scholar]

Chapter 16

ROLE OF PATHOLOGIST IN EMERGENCY SURGERY

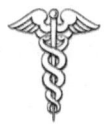

Dr Snigdha Goyal

Pathologists are medical specialists who have considerable skills which enable them to contribute significantly to the provision of high quality, efficient and effective health care. The skills they develop as a consequence of training, first as a medical practitioner, and then as a specialist pathologist, allow them to understand clinical disease processes and their diagnosis.

PATHOLOGIST

- Expert in clinical interpretation of diagnostic tests and an understanding of the nature and causation of disease processes

- Expert in understanding the principles of analysis and technical details of tests used to diagnose and monitor disease

- Expert in the development and assessment of new testing methodologies

- Expert in knowing the appropriate test to be performed: in a specific clinical situation ("the right test at the right time for the right patient")

- Expert in interpretation of individual and groups of test results and the significance these results will have on patient management

- Expert in quality methodologies in the laboratory

- Expert in safety requirements for laboratories

- Expert in the effect of disease and therapy on laboratory tests

ROLE OF PATHOLOGIST IN TREATMENT OF EMERGENCY PATIENTS

CBC Count

A complete blood count (CBC) is a blood test used to evaluate your overall health and detect a wide range of disorders, including anaemia, infection and leukaemia.

A complete blood count test measures several components and features of your blood, including:

- Red blood cells, which carry oxygen

- White blood cells, which fight infection

- Haemoglobin, the oxygen-carrying protein in red blood cells

- Haematocrit, the proportion of red blood cells to the fluid component, or plasma, in your blood

- Platelets, which help with blood clotting

Abnormal increases or decreases in cell counts as revealed in a complete blood count may indicate that you have an underlying medical condition that calls for further evaluation.

FROZEN SECTION

Intra-operative frozen section plays an important role in the management of surgical patients. The tissue specimen taken from a patient by doing a biopsy or an operation is usually assessed by the pathologist. Occasionally surgeons need pathologic information more urgently, thus they will request for an intra-operative consultation on the tissue that is being taken out.

The examination is made while the patient is under anaesthesia on the operating table. This involves gross inspection and, if it is a larger specimen, some dissection will be performed. Depending on the surgeon's inquiry and what the pathologist feels is necessary; a frozen section (FS) may be performed on the specimen and examined under the microscope. The examination report will then be conveyed as soon as possible to the operating surgeon via telephone or the intercom, and the result will greatly influence the surgeon's intra-operational decision.

FS may be one of the most important procedures performed by the pathologist during his practice. It is a difficult procedure. The pathologist has to arrive at a correct decision in a shorter duration under pressure, based on his experience, judgement and the knowledge of his specialty and clinical medicine. He should also have a keen awareness of the limitations of the method as the patient's life is often dramatically influenced by his report. Likewise, the operating surgeon should also realize the limitations of FS and it is imperative for him to make a prior appointment for FS and should always ask himself whether the results of the FS examination will in any way influence the surgical procedure. If the answer is no, then an FS examination is not indicated.[1]

The Modern Technique of Frozen Section

The development of a cryomicrotome, popularly known as cryostat in 1959, has revolutionized the FS technique. The cryostat is a refrigerated box containing a rotary microtome. The temperature inside the cryostat is about $-20°$ to $-30°$ Celsius. The attending technologist will then process the tissue section by freezing it with frozen aerosol sprays and put onto the cryostat for sectioning. Intra and intercellular water is frozen to produce a hard matrix to enable slicing of the tissue. The tissue sections are cut and picked up on glass slides, which are then ready for staining.

The overall impact of the cryostat was two-fold: (a) it made it possible to section quick-frozen, unfixed tissue in the 5–10 mm range of thickness and (b) the use of a modified H&E stain produced permanent preparation.

It takes about 5–10 minutes to prepare the slides. The time taken by the pathologist to study them under the microscope and arrive at a diagnosis is in addition to this.

In one study involving 700 laboratories worldwide, it was found that 90% of FS block turnaround times were within 20 minutes, measured from the time the pathologists received the FS specimens to the time that pathologists returned FS diagnoses to surgeons.[2]

Uses of Frozen Section

Both the surgeon and the pathologist should be fully aware of the indications for FS. This will allow the appropriate request to be attended to. As mentioned earlier, only those requests that will definitely influence intra-operative management should be duly entertained.

- i. Establish the nature of a lesion
- ii. Establish the presence of a lesion
- iii. Confirm the presence of a benign lesion
- iv. Confirm that sufficient tissue is present for diagnosis
- v. Establish the grade of the lesion
- vi. Determine the presence of synchronous lesions
- vii. Determine the organ of origin
- viii. Determine the adequacy of margins
- ix. Establish evidence of invasion
- x. Determine the presence of infection
- xi. Acquire fresh tissue for special studies

In a study done at the University of Michigan Hospitals, Ann Arbor, USA, on FS requests of 914 cases, it was noted that 95% were performed for appropriate reasons, which included evaluation of margins (46%), establishing a primary diagnosis (43%) and determining adequacy or viability of tissue (3%).[3]

Drawbacks

The limitations of FS need to be taken into consideration when requesting for this procedure, in order to avoid grave mistakes that will be detrimental to the patient's management. These limitations can be divided into three main categories namely sampling error, technical problem and interpretative error.[4]

Sampling slips or constraint:

   i. Poor sampling of tissue/limitation of the surgeons

   ii. Poor selection of appropriate tissue after grossing

   iii. Extensive tumour degeneration or necrosis

   iv. Poor assessment of capsular or vascular invasion

   v. Malignant component in ovarian teratoma

Searching for an immature component in an ovarian teratoma is rather time consuming in FS and subject to sampling error. It is not possible for all the tumours to be sampled either intra-operatively or in the pathology laboratory for FS. Therefore, a report of benign teratoma does not totally rule out a malignant one until the tumour is adequately sampled later.

Technical Problems

   i. Freezing artifacts/Xylene artifacts

   ii. Poor quality section

   iii. Bloated cell morphology

   iv. Poorly stained section

Interpretative Errors

FS diagnosis sometimes can be very tricky. It is the policy of the pathologist to give the closest diagnosis as possible to the surgeon and avoid giving a definitive diagnosis if there is any doubt. It is preferable to delay the definitive diagnosis of the case, especially if the finding(s) is not going to influence the intra-operative management.

These are some of the difficulties that may be encountered in FS service:

i. Tumours that are difficult to diagnose

ii. Heterogeneity of the tumour

iii. Mixed tumour and biphasic tumour

iv. Variable degrees of tumour differentiation

v. Difficult assessment of chronic pancreatitis versus pancreatic carcinoma

vi. Difficulty in assessing ganglion cells and hypertrophied nerve bundles in Hirschsprung disease

CLOSE COOPERATION AND RAPPORT BETWEEN SURGEON AND PATHOLOGIST

Close cooperation between the surgeon and the pathologist is required if a meaningful frozen report is to be achieved. Preferably, the case should be discussed beforehand between the surgeon and the pathologist. The pathologist should not be treated as a mere technician, and all the relevant information must be conveyed to him for the benefit of the patient.

The pathologist must be prepared and have a high suspicion index.

The pathologist should attend the FS fully prepared which includes reading the literature about the suspected tumour and the possible histological variants and grading. With the relevant clinical information, the pathologist should have a high index of suspicion and look for the histological features concerned.

The pathologist should have the final say.

The pathologist should be party to the decision of whether or not a FS should be done. After taking into consideration the reason(s) for FS, the clinical presentation of the case, and all relevant investigations done on the patient, the pathologist should decide whether the FS is worth pursuing. If not, then it is wise and safe to wait for a proper histopathological report of the case rather than trying to make an unreasonable diagnosis that may have dire consequences for the patient.

REFERENCES

1. Hasnan Jaafar. Intra-Operative Frozen Section Consultation: Concepts, Applications and Limitations Malays J Med Sci. 2006 Jan; 13(1): 4–12.

2. David AN, Richard JZ. Inter-institutional comparison of frozen section turnaround time. Archives of Pathology & Laboratory Medicine. 1997;121(6):559–68. [PubMed]

3. Weiss SW, Willis J, Jansen J, Goldblum J, Greenfield L. Frozen section consultation. Utilization patterns and knowledge base of surgical faculty at a university hospital. Am J Clin Pathol. 1995;104(3):294–8.[PubMed]

4. Ackerman LV, Ramirez GA. The indications for and limitations of frozen section diagnosis: A review of 1269 consecutive frozen sections. Br J Surg. 1959;46:336. [PubMed]

Chapter 17

ROLE OF EMERGENCY DIAGNOSTIC LAPAROSCOPY IN ACUTE ABDOMEN

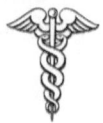

Parveen Bhatia

Laparoscopy is a minimal-access surgical procedure that allows visual examination of diseases of all intra-abdominal organs with the help of laparoscopy. Diagnostic laparoscopy was first introduced in 1901, when the German surgeon, Georg Kelling performed a "peritoneoscopy" on a dog, which was termed, "celioscopy". Diagnostic laparoscopy on humans was done for the assessment of ascites in 1910. Emergency diagnostic laparoscopy was first proposed by Philippe Moment in 1990.

Acute nonspecific abdominal pain is generally defined as 'acute abdominal pain' when it lasts less than seven days, and for which there is no diagnosis after examination and baseline investigations. Abdominal pain may occur due to simple disease or it may arise from a life-threatening ailment, needing immediate surgery.

The abdomen is a Pandora's box of diagnostic dilemma. It is obligatory on the part of a surgeon to diagnose the pain and decide whether to operate immediately, treat it conservatively, or to observe the patient. The surgeon has to be very careful regarding proper diagnosis and treatment due to medicolegal litigation, also.

Emergency surgery is required in acute appendicitis, perforation, ovarian torsion, ectopic pregnancy and rupture. Acute abdominal pain represents 1% of hospital admissions and 6% of emergency cases. Proper history, physical examination, laboratory and radiological tests can diagnose most of the diseases. However, in some cases it is not possible to reach a final diagnosis. It is a significant problem in general surgery and accounts for an estimated 13% to 40% of emergency surgical admissions.

Despite new diagnostic developments like ultrasonography and computed tomography, sometimes an acute abdominal condition presents a situation, in which the surgeon has to perform a laparotomy which may be negative, and adds unnecessary morbidity to the patient. Such patients, with unclear diagnosis, are admitted and put under active clinical observation ("wait and watch"). The predictive value of clinical diagnosis reached by this method is 68% to 92%. A delay in surgical intervention may increase morbidity and prolong hospital stay. Clinical observation could lead to an overall higher cost of treatment and radiation exposure - due to repeated radiological tests, more antibiotic and analgesic requirement, and a longer hospital stay. Therefore, early presentation to the hospital and early intervention through diagnostic laparoscopy in such cases, can prevent further morbidity and mortality, and improve the patient's satisfaction and quality of life.

Diagnostic laparoscopy is useful for making a definitive clinical diagnosis whenever there is a diagnostic dilemma. Laparoscopy reveals either no abnormality or discovers a disease that does not require surgery for proper management, thus avoiding the unnecessary burden of non-therapeutic laparotomies. Laparoscopy is particularly useful in women of childbearing age in whom tubo-ovarian abnormality simulates acute appendicitis. Without laparoscopy, the overall rate of unnecessary appendectomy is high.

Diagnostic laparoscopy has ample advantages over conventional investigations like ultrasound and even laparotomy. Diagnostic laparoscopy allows visualisation of pelvic and para-colic gutters which can't be seen on laparotomy. Diagnostic laparoscopy has proved a boon for dubious clinical diagnoses, and negative laparotomies can be easily prevented. It reduces the rate of negative and nontherapeutic laparotomies (with a subsequent decrease in hospitalization, morbidity, and cost, after negative laparoscopy). In patients who are under observation, it helps in early diagnosis and early management.

Diagnostic laparoscopy offers many advantages in the management of many intra-abdominal conditions where the correct diagnosis could not be established clinically, or even after radiological tests. In most of the patients, the clinical signs and symptoms are masked by the treatments given by the different physicians at different hospitals at different points of time. Also, by different radiologists giving different reports of imaging studies that have to be correlated clinically. In these circumstances, diagnostic laparoscopy alone helps solve the issue.

Diagnostic laparoscopy reduces the number of negative laparotomies in acute abdomen and prevents severe peritonitis which may occur as a result of delay in diagnosis. Diagnostic laparoscopy plays an important role in the evaluation of abdominal pain in young children. Mesenteric ischemia and the subsequent bowel gangrene can be better controlled and managed reasonably if early diagnostic laparoscopy is advocated.

Computer-aided diagnostic questionnaires, abdominal ultrasound (US), abdominal computed tomography (CT) scan, and early laparoscopy have all been described as potential methods for improving diagnosis. Laparoscopy is the most effective technique for bridging the gap between clinical evaluation and major surgical exploration. Advantages in terms of safety, reduced morbidity and mortality, decreased postoperative pain and short hospital stay makes it a valuable diagnostic tool.

The overall diagnostic rate is 99% for acute abdominal pain, 70% for chronic pain syndrome, 95% for focal liver disorders, 95% for abdominal masses, 95% for ascites and 80% for retroperitoneal disease. Diagnostic accuracy of laparoscopy in abdominal trauma is 91%, and laparotomy is found unnecessary in 54% of patients. Incorporation of diagnostic laparoscopy along with biopsy, may improve the management of vague abdominal pain, by making a definite diagnosis, access for immediate treatment, reducing hospital stay and readmission rates and, eventually, having cost benefits. Diagnostic laparoscopy has a sensitivity and specificity of 100%.

REFERENCES

1. Thomas A, Stellate MD: History of Laparoscopic Surgery. Surg Clin North Am 1992; 72:997-1002.

2. Cuschieri A. and Buess G: Introduction and historical aspects: Operative manual of endoscopic surgery. Springer-verlag. 1992.

3. Subramaniam R. Diagnostic laparoscopy in acute abdominal pain. Int Surg J. 2019 Apr; 6 (4):1104-1107.

4. Anand Thawait, Sankalp Dwivedi, Manisha Bhatt, Karan Bakhshish, Amit Mittal. Role of early laparoscopy in diagnosis of acute abdominal pain. International Journal of Contemporary Medical Research 2017;4(7):1568-1574.

5. Ahmed MM, Dar HM, Waseem M, et.al. Role of laparoscopy in nonspecific abdominal pain. Saudi Surg J[serial online] 2014[cited 2020 Jan 19]; 2: 71-4.

Chapter 18

COMMON UROLOGY EMERGENCY

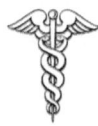

Nishant Gurnani

A urology emergency refers to any urologic condition that requires urgent medical attention along with GU trauma. Few urologic problems are considered emergencies, so the list is limited to only a handful of conditions. These conditions, when left untreated, are potentially life-threatening or may result in serious long-term complications or consequences.

"Urologic trauma" is the term used to describe extreme damage to the genitourinary system and can be caused by an automobile accident, gunshot wound, or any other act of violence.

As compared to other surgical specialties, urological emergencies are few and can be divided as follows:

NON-TRAUMATIC UROLOGICAL EMERGENCIES

1. Retention of urine

2. Hematuria

3. Renal colic

4. Acute scrotum

5. Priapism

6. Paraphimosis

7. Fournier's gangrene

TRAUMATIC UROLOGICAL EMERGENCIES

1. Renal trauma

2. Bladder trauma

3. Urethral trauma

4. Penile trauma

NON-TRAUMATIC UROLOGICAL EMERGENCIES

1. Retention of Urine

Definition:

Acute retention of urine: Painful, palpable or percussible bladder, when the patient is unable to pass any urine [1]

Chronic retention of urine: Non-painful bladder, which remains palpable or percussible after the patient has passed urine. Such patients may be incontinent [1].

Bladder outlet obstruction (BOO): Generic term for obstruction during voiding, characterized by increasing detrusor pressure and reduced urine flow rate.

Benign prostatic obstruction (BPO): A form of BOO which may be diagnosed when the cause of outlet obstruction is known to be Benign Prostatic Enlargement (BPE).

Causes for retention of urine:

Men	Women	Both
Benign Prostatic Obstruction	Pelvic Prolapse (cystocele/ rectocele/uterine)	Blood clot
Urethral stricture	Post-surgery for stress incontinence	Neurogenic bladder (Diabetes/spinal cord injury)
Phimosis	Pelvic masses	Urethral calculus
Acute urethritis/ prostatitis	Bladder neck stricture (Rare)	Faecal impaction
		Anal pain
		Drugs (Anticholinergics)
		Spinal anaesthesia

Management: Placement of per urethral or supra pubic catheter

Post catheterization, monitor the patient vitals and urine output. Patients with long standing obstructive uropathy (azotemia with obstruction in urinary tract) may have post obstructive diuresis.

Post obstructive diuresis is defined as urine output of more than 200 ml/hour. If the patient has post obstructive diuresis, monitor vitals strictly, replace fluid with intravenous saline equal to urine output per hour and get 12 hourly serum electrolytes. Specialized management by a urologist is necessary in such cases.

2. Haematuria

Haematuria is a frightening diagnosis both, for the patient, and the physician. As such, any incidence of haematuria, during any part of life, is significant and should be evaluated, however late may be the presentation.

Definitions:

Microscopic haematuria: More than 3RBC/HPF, variety of causes like stone, cancer of bladder, upper urinary tract, UTI

Gross haematuria: Haematuria visible to naked eye, most commonly due to bladder cancer or transitional cell cancer of kidney

Initial haematuria: Haematuria during the starting of voiding which clears later; causes include urethral pathology

Terminal haematuria: Haematuria during the end of voiding; causes include pathology of prostatic urethra or bladder neck

Total haematuria: Haematuria throughout the course of voiding; causes include bladder or upper urinary tract pathology

Per urethral bleed: Bleeding from the meatus unrelated to voiding, variety of causes

Work Up:

a. History and physical examination: Identify severity of current episode in terms of duration, presence of clots, lower urinary tract symptoms. Identify previous incidences of haematuria/ previous interventions/use of anticoagulants/ smoking status/intake of drugs

b. Haemogram with PT/INR: To look for current haemoglobin and coagulation status and also for drop in haemoglobin if continuing haematuria for definitive treatment

c. Renal function test with serum electrolytes: To look for upper tract pathology

d. USG KUB with prostate: Look for pathology (stone/mass) in kidney and bladder, presence of clots in bladder

e. CECT Scan: Should be done in all cases of gross haematuria - to look for the same pathology as in USG

f. Cystoscopy: Diagnostic after the patient is stable. Therapeutic with fulguration of bleeding points in cases with continuing haematuria and drop in haemoglobin.

Management:

1. Stabilize the patient

2. Intravenous fluids

3. Insert 22 Fr three-way Foley's catheter and start NS irrigation through 3rd channel at rate of 300–400 ml/hour

4. Monitor for clearing for haematuria

5. If haematuria clears slow the irrigation rate to 100 ml/hour for 4–6 hours and then finally stop. Then evaluate patient for cause of haematuria

6. If haematuria continues with drop in haemoglobin then do cystoscopy with trans-urethral fulguration of bleeding points and clot removal

Haemorrhagic cystitis

It is characterised by diffuse inflammation and bleeding from bladder mucosa.

Causes of haemorrhagic cystitis:[2]

- Infectious: Bacterial, BK virus, adenovirus

- Trauma

- Malignancy: Primary bladder cancer or invasion from surrounding structures

- Chemical exposure: Cyclophosphamide, dyes, ethers

- Post radiation therapy

Management of haemorrhagic cystitis:

See Fig 1. Below

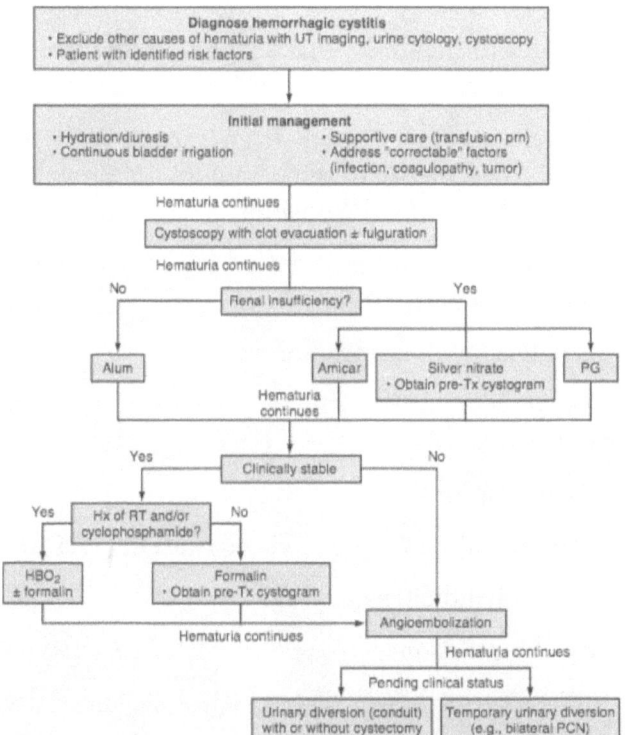

Fig 1: Management of haemorrhagic cystitis HBO2, hyperbaric oxygen, Hx history, PCN percutaneous nephrostomy, PG prostaglandin, Tx treatment; UT upper tract. Adapted from Campbell Walsh Urology 11th edition 2016.

3. Renal Colic

It is one of the commonest causes of "Acute Abdomen". Sudden onset of severe pain in the flank, most often due to the passage of a stone formed in the kidney, down through the ureter.

The pain is characterized by:

- very sudden onset
- colicky in nature
- Radiates to the groin as the stone passes into the lower ureter.
- May change in location, from the flank to the groin, (the location of the pain does not provide a good indication of the position of the stone)
- The patient cannot get comfortable, and may roll around in agony.
- Associated with nausea/vomiting.

  "The pain of passing a ureteric stone as bad as the pain of labour"

Differential diagnosis:

- Ovarian pathology (e.g., twisted ovarian cyst)
- Acute appendicitis
- Testicular torsion
- Inflammatory bowel disease (Crohn's, ulcerative colitis)
- Diverticulitis
- Ectopic pregnancy
- Burst peptic ulcer
- Bowel obstruction

Work up:

- History
- Examination: patient continually moves around in an attempt to find a comfortable position

- Pregnancy test

- Urine R/M and culture

Radiological Investigations:

- KUB/Abdominal US

- X ray KUB

- Helical CTU [3]

  ➤ Greater specificity (95%) and sensitivity (97%) for diagnosing ureteric stones than IVU

  ➤ Can identify other, non-stone causes of flank pain

  ➤ No need for contrast administration

  ➤ Faster, taking just a few minutes

Acute Management of Ureteric Stones:

1. Pain relief with NSAIDs: Intramuscular or intravenous injection, by mouth, or per rectum.

   No relief with NSAIDS: Opiate analgesics (pethidine or morphine).

2. Hyper hydration: No role.

3. Medical expulsive therapy: Tamsulosin 0.4 mg has an off-label use [4] in promoting expulsion of ureteral stones and to relax the ureter during a colic episode. Similar role of corticosteroids and calcium channel blockers like nifedipine has been studied, but their efficacy is still not yet proven.

Indications for Intervention to Relieve Obstruction and/ or Remove the Stone:

1. Pain that fails to respond to analgesics

2. Presence of urosepsis

3. Renal function is impaired because of the stone (solitary kidney obstructed by a stone, bilateral ureteric stones, or pre-existing renal impairment)

4. Failure of Medical Expulsive Therapy

5. Personal or occupational reasons

Treatment of the Stone:

- Temporary relief of the obstruction:
  - ➤ Insertion of a JJ stent or percutaneous nephrostomy tube

- Definitive treatment of stone:
  - ➤ ESWL
  - ➤ PCNL
  - ➤ Ureteroscopy
  - ➤ Open Surgery (very limited)

4. Acute Scrotum

Emergency situation requiring prompt evaluation, differential diagnosis, and potentially immediate surgical exploration.

Differential Diagnosis:

- Torsion of spermatic cord: Most serious

- Torsion of appendix testis

- Torsion of epididymis

- Epididymitis: Most common

- Epididymo-orchitis

- Inguinal hernia

- Communicating hydrocele

- Hydrocele of cord

- Varicocele

- Spermatocele

- Inflammatory vasculitis

Torsion of spermatic cord [5,6,7]

- Intravaginal torsion predisposed by bell clapper deformity; tunica vaginalis fixed abnormally proximal to cord

- May occur at any age but peaks between 12–16 years

- History of prior episodes elicited

- Physical findings: generalized testicular tenderness, abnormal horizontal orientation of testis, absent cremasteric reflex

- Colour Doppler USG is 86% sensitive, 100% specific, and 97% accurate in the diagnosis of torsion [8]

Management of testicular torsion

- True surgical emergency of the highest order [9]

- Irreversible ischemic injury to the testicular parenchyma may begin as soon as **hours**

- Testicular salvage decreases as duration of torsion increases, risk orchiectomy 90% after more than 48 hours of onset of pain [10]

- Testicular atrophy may occur even after surgical detorsion within four hours of onset of pain [10]

- Manual detorsion may not completely untwist the cord [10]

- Surgical exploration:

  ➤ Median raphe incision

  ➤ Explore affected side first

  ➤ Untwist the cord

  ➤ Place warm sponges on testis and assess for viability with incision on tunica albuginea, return of pink color, or color Doppler

  ➤ If testis viable, sartos suture fixation with non-absorbable suture

  ➤ If testis not viable; orchiectomy done

  ➤ Suture fix contralateral testis to prevent further detorsion

Prognosis:

- Impact on fertility poorly understood

- Semen density may be poor in long duration torsion [11]

Epididymo-orchitis:

- Presentation

  ➤ Indolent process

➤ Scrotal swelling, erythema, and pain

➤ Dysuria and fever are more common

- Physical examination

  ➤ localized epididymal tenderness, a swollen and tender epididymis, or a massively swollen hemiscrotum with absence of landmarks

  ➤ Cremasteric reflex should be present

- Urine:

  ➤ Pyuria, bacteriuria, or a positive urine culture (Gram-negative bacteria)

- Imaging

  ➤ In a prepubertal child with a positive urine culture, renal ultrasonography and voiding cysto-urethrography are indicated

- Management

  ➤ Bed rest for 1–3 days, then relative restriction

  ➤ Scrotal elevation, the use of an athletic supporter

  ➤ Parenteral antibiotic therapy should be instituted when UTI is documented or suspected

  ➤ Urethral instrumentation should be avoided

5. Priapism

- Persistent erection of the penis for more than four hours that is not related to, or accompanied by, sexual desire [2].

- Two Types:

  ➤ Ischaemic (veno-occlusive, low flow (most common)

    ◦ Due to haematological disease, malignant infiltration of the corpora cavernosa with malignant disease, or drugs

    ◦ Painful

  ➤ Non-ischaemic (arterial, high flow)

    ◦ Due to perineal trauma, which creates an arteriovenous fistula

    ◦ Painless

- Age:

  ➤ Any age

  ➤ Two main age groups affected are 5 to 10-year-old boys and 20 to 50-year-old men

- Causes:

  ➤ Primary (Idiopathic): 30%- 50%

  ➤ Secondary:

    ◦ Drugs

    ◦ Trauma

    ◦ Neurological

    ◦ Hematological disease

    ◦ Tumors

    ◦ Miscellaneous

- Diagnosis:
  - ➤ Usually obvious from the history
    - ○ Duration of erection >4 hours?
    - ○ Is it painful or not?
    - ○ Previous history and treatment of priapism?
    - ○ Identify any predisposing factors and underlying causes
- Examination:
  - ➤ Erect, tender penis (in low-flow priapism)
  - ➤ Characteristically the corpora cavernosa is rigid and the glans is flaccid
  - ➤ Abdomen, for evidence of malignant disease
  - ➤ DRE: to examine the prostate and check anal tone
- Investigations:
  - ➤ CBC (white cell count and differential, reticulocyte count)
  - ➤ Hemoglobin electrophoresis for sickle cell test
  - ➤ Urinalysis including urine toxicology
  - ➤ Color flow duplex ultrasonography in cavernosal arteries:
    - ○ Ischaemic (inflow low or nonexistent)
    - ○ Non-ischaemic (inflow normal to high).

➤ Blood gases taken from either corpora:

○ **low-flow** (dark blood; pH <7.25 (acidosis); pO2 <30 mm Hg (hypoxia); pCO2 >60 mm Hg (hypercapnia))

○ **high-flow** (bright red blood similar to arterial blood at room temperature; pH = 7.4; pO2 >90 mm Hg; pCO2 <40 mm Hg)

➤ Penile pudendal arteriography: in suspected cases of penile trauma to diagnose high flow priapism

• Treatment [12]:

➤ Depends on the type of priapism

➤ Conservative treatment should first be tried

Medical treatment:

• Ischemic priapism: decompression of corpora cavernosa with aspiration of blood +/- corporal phenylephrine injections (as 200 ug/ml up to a maximum dose of 1 mg)

• No role of oral drugs for ischemic priapism

• Aspiration continued till no more dark blood aspirated and fresh red bright blood is obtained

• Non-ischaemic priapism not an emergency, spontaneous resolution seen in 62% cases, treatment is selective arterial embolization

• Surgical treatment: in non-resolving cases of ischemic priapism, shunt made between corpora cavernosa with either glans/corpora spongiosum/ dorsal penile vein

6. Paraphimosis

This condition results due to forceful reduction of tight prepuce in uncircumcised males. The foreskin of the penis becomes swollen and inflamed. The inflammation may cause the foreskin to compress on the glans thus impairing proper blood flow and causing the swelling to worsen. It primarily occurs in adolescents and senior men who require frequent catheterizations. Treatment is primarily geared towards bringing the swelling down, then repairing the foreskin or putting it back over the glans. If oedema cannot be reduced and prepuce cannot be brought forward then the patient needs urgent dorsal slit or circumcision, because, when left untreated, paraphimosis can lead to tissue death in the penis and, eventually, to gangrene.

7. Fournier's Gangrene

With an almost 50% fatality rate [13], Fournier's Gangrene is an infection of the genitals that rapidly progresses, causing tissue death and thus requiring emergency treatment. It is usually caused by mixed bacterial flora, including gram positive, gram negative and anaerobic bacteria. The infection spreads along the fascial planes and hence the exterior appearance of skin may underestimate the spread of infection The infection may stem from a variety of root causes, but susceptibility to it has been linked to steroid use, excessive alcohol consumption, and even underlying diseases such as diabetes.

Symptoms linked with this condition include redness, swelling, and extreme pain in the scrotum or perineum which is out of proportion to physical findings. Some may also have fever and chills. Treatment involves broad spectrum antibiotics with extensive surgical debridation till the point of healthy bleeding is seen. Usually the testis can be spared even in extensive infections [14]. Role of hyperbaric oxygen therapy is controversial [15]. Vacuum assisted closure devices help in early resolution of infection [16]. Patients may need a urinary diversion in the form of supra pubic catheter in cases of urethral involvement and to prevent soiling of wound. Most patients have some form of sexual dysfunction of up to 65% [17].

TRAUMATIC UROLOGICAL EMERGENCIES

1. Renal Trauma

Most renal injuries (85 to 90% of cases) result from blunt trauma, typically due to motor vehicle crashes, falls, or assaults. Most injuries are low grade. The most common accompanying injuries are to the head, central nervous system, chest, spleen, and liver. Penetrating injuries usually result from gunshot wounds and are usually associated with multiple, intra-abdominal injuries, most commonly to the chest, liver, intestine, and spleen.

Renal injuries are classified by severity into five grades (American Association for the Surgery of Trauma, 2018 revision), based on CECT findings, and is highly predictive of outcomes:

- Grade 1: Subcapsular hematoma and/or renal contusion

- Grade 2: Laceration ≤ 1 cm in depth without urinary extravasation

- Grade 3: Laceration > 1 cm without urinary extravasation

- Grade 4: Laceration involving the collecting system with urinary extravasation; any segmental renal vascular injury; renal infarction; renal pelvis laceration and/or ureteropelvic disruption

- Grade 5: Shattered or devascularized kidney with active bleeding; main renal vascular laceration or avulsion

Presentation and History [2]:

It is important to elicit the extent of deceleration in blunt trauma as the kidney is susceptible to injury at the points of fixation in retroperitoneum, such as renal hilum and ureteropelvic junction.

Gunshot wounds are more liable to cause penetrating injuries as compared to stab wounds. Penetrating injuries of kidney are associated with higher rates of delayed nephrectomy if managed conservatively. Trauma in the anterior axillary line is more prone to damage the renovascular structures while trauma along the posterior axillary line commonly involves the parenchyma.

Best indicators of urinary system injury include gross or microscopic haematuria, however the degree of haematuria does not correlate with severity of injury.

Indications for renal imaging [2]

1. All stable patients with a penetrating injury, with a likelihood of renal injury (abdomen, flank, or low chest entry/exit wound)

2. All blunt trauma patients with significant deceleration as would occur in high speed motor vehicle or fall from height

3. All blunt trauma with gross haematuria

4. All blunt trauma with microscopic haematuria and with hypotension

5. All paediatric patients with microscopic haematuria

Contrast enhanced CT scan is the imaging of choice for renal trauma [18]. Findings on CT scan like medial haematoma, medial urinary extravasation and global lack of contrast enhancement of kidney are suggestive of renal injury.

There is a limited role for an intraoperative, one shot IVP. It is basically done when the surgeon unexpectedly encounters a kidney injury in a patient with no previous CT scan. It helps in assessing the presence of a normal contralateral kidney, and if the injured kidney is the sole functioning unit in the patient, then an attempt must be made to repair it.

Patients who are taking anticoagulants or who have a congenital renal anomaly can develop gross haematuria after relatively minor trauma.

Treatment:

• Strict bed rest with close monitoring of vital signs

• Surgical repair or angiographic intervention for some blunt and most penetrating high-grade renal injuries

Most blunt renal injuries, including all grade 1 and 2 and most grade 3 and 4 injuries, can be safely managed non-operatively. Patients should be maintained on strict bed rest until the gross haematuria has resolved. Intervention is required for patients with the following:

- Hemodynamic instability

- Expanding perinephric haematoma

- Renal pedicle avulsion or other significant renovascular injuries

Intervention can include surgery, stent placement, or selective angiographic embolization.

Penetrating trauma usually requires surgical exploration, although observation may be appropriate for patients in whom the renal injury has been accurately staged by CT, blood pressure is stable, and no associated intra-abdominal injuries require surgery.

2. Bladder Injury

Bladder perforations may be traumatic or spontaneous in origin. The majority of bladder injuries are due to trauma. Trauma can be blunt , penetrating, or iatrogenic. Blunt and penetrating trauma to the bladder are accompanied with pelvic fracture or a gunshot wound to the pelvis [19]. Iatrogenic causes of injury include pelvic surgery, suprapubic or urethral placement of a Foley catheter (especially a long-term indwelling catheter), bladder biopsy, and ureteral stent manipulation. Injury can be extra peritoneal or intraperitoneal. Bladder rupture does not occur as an isolated, asymptomatic event in normal individuals. Conscious patients present with pronounced nonspecific symptoms -such as suprapubic pain combined with an inability to void.

Imaging of the bladder is performed on the basis of clinical suspicion. After blunt external trauma, the absolute indication for immediate cystography is gross haematuria associated with pelvic fracture. Plain film cystography or CT cystography with retrograde filling of bladder with contrast are investigations of choice [20].

A dense, flame-shaped collection of contrast material in the pelvis is characteristic of extra peritoneal extravasation. Depending on fascial integrity, contrast material may extend beyond the confines of the pelvis and be visualized in the retro peritoneum, scrotum, phallus, thigh, or abdominal wall. The amount of extravasation is not always proportional to the extent of bladder injury. Intraperitoneal extravasation is identified when contrast material outlines loops of bowel and/or the lower lateral portion of the peritoneal cavity.

Bladder tears can be divided as extra peritoneal, intraperitoneal, or combined. Extra peritoneal bladder tears constitute approximately 80%–90% of all bladder tears and are associated with pelvic fractures that cause perforation of the bladder wall. The usual treatment of uncomplicated extra peritoneal bladder ruptures, when conditions are ideal, is conservative management with urethral catheter drainage alone. A large-bore (22-Fr) Foley catheter should be used to promote adequate drainage; if output is poor, fluoroscopic cystography should be considered to ensure proper catheter placement. Cystography is necessary to verify complete healing before catheter removal 14 days after injury. Antimicrobial agents are instituted on the day of injury and continued for at least one week to prevent infection of the pelvic haematoma.

Intraperitoneal bladder tears account for approximately 10%–20% of bladder injuries and occur at the dome of the distended bladder, which is the only part that is covered by the peritoneum. Intraperitoneal perforations result in a communication between the urinary bladder and the peritoneal cavity, with resultant extravasation of contrast solution into the paracolic gutters or the rectovesical or recto uterine pouch or around multiple loops of bowel. Intraperitoneal bladder tears often require surgical intervention [21].

Indications for immediate repair of bladder injury

- Intraperitoneal injury from external trauma

- Penetrating or iatrogenic non-urologic injury

- Inadequate bladder drainage or clots in urine

- Bladder neck injury

- Rectal or vaginal injury

- Open pelvic fracture

- Pelvic fracture requiring open reduction and internal fixation

- Selected stable patients undergoing laparotomy for other reasons

- Bone fragments projecting into bladder

3. Urethral Injury

Urethral injury is a breach in the structural integrity of the urethra resulting from excessive trauma. The incidence of urethral injury is on the rise due to increasing industrialization and high-speed commutes.

Accurate diagnosis is necessary for appropriate acute management and reduction of long-term morbidity.

Classification

- Posterior urethral injury
- Anterior urethral injury

Aetiology of posterior urethral injury

- Part of multisystem trauma
- Pelvic fracture involving all four pubic rami has highest risk of injury [22]
- Pelvic fracture - 10% associated with urethral injury
- Bulbo-membranous junction most vulnerable [23]
- Urethral sphincter remains intact [24]

Aetiology of anterior urethral injury

- Anterior urethral injury (usually isolated)
- Straddle injury – injury occurs in bulbar urethra
- Iatrogenic – catheter-related – bouginage – endoscopy – mechanical or electrical – circumcision – penetrating injury – gunshot – penile fracture – self-mutilation – mentally ill – sexual gratification
- Female urethra: Pelvic fracture/vaginal surgery

Diagnosis [25]

- Triad of blood at meatus, inability to urinate and palpable bladder

- Other classic findings: high riding prostate/ butterfly perineal haematoma

- Inability to pass a urethral catheter, usually the first sign in absence of above findings

- Urethrography : retrograde urethrography should be performed immediately in presence of above findings

Initial management

- Immediate open reconstruction: Abandoned in males, in view of increased incidence of stricture, impotence and blood loss [26]. Some authorities advocate primary realignment in females to avoid fistula formation [27]

- Suprapubic cystostomy: standard of care in men with posterior urethral injury

- Primary realignment: Not routinely recommended but may be done after a few days of injury in stable patients preferably under endoscopic vision [28].

Delayed reconstruction

- Placement of SPC leads to scar formation at injury site, which is complete by three months

- MCU and RGU are done to assess stricture length

- Posterior urethroplasty or endoscopic treatment may then be undertaken, provided other injuries have healed and patient is ambulatory [29].

Follow Up

- Peri-catheter study is done at two weeks to rule out extravasation of dye from anastomotic site

- If no leak then SPC is clamped and urethral catheter is removed, followed by SPC removal after two weeks

- Complications include: erectile dysfunction (50%) [30], recurrent stricture (5–15%) [31], incontinence (4%) [32]

4. Trauma to Penis

Penile Fracture [33,34,35]

A penile fracture can occur during sexual intercourse or vigorous masturbation when an erect penis is bent forcibly. However, penile fractures may also be the result of blunt trauma inflicted on the erect penis. Penile fractures occur due to the disruption of the tunica albuginea with rupture of corpora cavernosa.

Signs of a penile fracture include immediate pain, instant erection loss, and a popping sensation. This is followed by swelling of the penis known as "eggplant deformity." Those suffering from a penile fracture may also experience pain when urinating and haematuria if the urethra was also damaged.

Diagnosis is with history and examination alone. In cases with suspected urethral injury, preoperative urethrography/urethroscopy may be done.

Treatment for penile fractures involve immediate surgery to close the tear where the penis is ruptured. The primary goal of treatment is to restore patient's urinary function and the ability to achieve erections.

Zipper injuries [36,37,38]

These are common among impatient boys and intoxicated men. Multiple manoeuvres are available to free the entrapped skin and to remove the mechanism. After a penile block, the zipper slider and adjacent skin can be lubricated with mineral oil, followed by a single attempt to unzip and untangle the skin. The cloth material connected to the zipper can be incised with perpendicular cuts in between each zipper tooth to release the lateral support of the zipper, allowing the device to fall apart and release the trapped skin. A bone cutter or similar tool can be used to cut the median bar (diamond-shaped connection) of the slider.

REFERENCES

1. Abrams, P., et al. The standardization of terminology of lower urinary tract function: report from the Standardization Sub-committee of the International Continence Society. Neurourol Urodyn, 2002. 21: 167.

2. Campbell-Walsh urology/editor-in-chief, Alan J. Wein ; editors, Louis R. Kavoussi ... [et al.]. 10th ed. c2012.

3. Smith RC, Rosen eld AT, Choe KA, et al. Acute ank pain: comparison of non-contrast-enhanced CT and intravenous urography. Radiology 1995; 194:789–94.

4. Kupeli B, Irkilata L, Gurocak S, et al. Does Tamsulosin enhance lower ureteral stone clearance with or without shock wave lithotripsy? Urology 2004;64(6):1111–5.

5. Williamson RC. Torsion of the testis and allied conditions. Br J Surg 1976;63:465–76.

6. Mushtaq I, Fung M, Glasson MJ. Retrospective review of paediatric patients with acute scrotum. Aust N Z J Surg 2003;73:55–8.

7. Cubillos J, Palmer JS, Friedman SC, et al. Familial testicular torsion. J Urol 2011;185(6 Suppl.):2469–72.

8. Burks DD, Markey BJ, Burkhard TK, et al. Suspected testicular torsion and ischemia: evaluation with color Doppler sonography. Radiology 1990; 175:815–21.

9. Visser AJ, Heyns CF. Testicular function after torsion of the spermatic cord. BJU Int 2003;92:200–3.

10. Sessions AE, Rabinowitz R, Hulbert WC, et al. Testicular torsion: direction, degree, duration and disinformation. J Urol 2003;169:663–5.

11. Arap MA, Vicentini FC, Cocuzza M, et al. Late hormonal levels, semen parameters, and presence of antisperm antibodies in patients treated for testicular torsion. J Androl 2007;28:528–32.

12. Montague DK, Jarow J, Broderick GA, et al. American Urological Association guideline on the management of priapism. J Urol 2003;170:1318–24.

13. Dahm P, Roland FH, Vaslef SN, et al. Outcome analysis in patients with primary necrotizing fasciitis of the male genitalia. Urology 2000;56:31–5, discussion 35–6.

14. Gurdal M, Yucebas E, Tekin A, et al. Predisposing factors and treatment outcome in Fournier's gangrene. Analysis of 28 cases. Urol Int 2003;70: 286–90.

15. Eke N. Fournier's gangrene: a review of 1726 cases. Br J Surg 2000;87: 718–28.

16. Czymek R, Schmidt A, Eckmann C, et al. Fournier's gangrene: vacuum- assisted closure versus conventional dressings. Am J Surg 2009;197: 168–76.

17. Czymek R, Kujath P, Bruch HP, et al. Treatment, outcome and quality of life after Fournier's gangrene: a multi-centre study. Colorectal Dis 2013;15: 1529–36.

18. Federle MP, Brown TR, McAninch JW. Penetrating renal trauma: CT evaluation. J Comp Assist Tomogr 1987;11:1026–30.

19. Bjurlin MA, Fantus RJ, Mellett MM, et al. Genitourinary injuries in pelvic fracture morbidity and mortality using the National Trauma Data Bank. J Trauma 2009;67:1033–9.

20. Peng MY, Parisky YR, Cornwell EE III, et al. CT cystography versus conventional cystography in evaluation of bladder injury. AJR Am J Roentgenol 1999;173:1269–72.

21. Deibert CM, Spencer BA. The association between operative repair of bladder injury and improved survival: results from the National Trauma Data Bank. J Urol 2011;186:151–5

22. Mundy AR. Urethroplasty for posterior urethral strictures. Br J Urol 1996;78:243-7.

23. Colapinto V, McCallum RW. Injury to the male posterior urethra in fractured pelvis: a new classification. J Urol 1977;118:575-80.

24. Andrich DE, Mundy AR. The nature of urethral injury in cases of pelvic fracture urethral trauma. J Urol 2001;165:1492-5.

25. Sandler CM, Corriere JN Jr. Urethrography in the diagnosis of acute urethral injuries. Urol Clin North Am 1989;16:283-9.

26. Webster GD, Mathes GL, Selli C. Prostatomembranous urethral injuries: a review of the literature and a rational approach to their management. J Urol 1983;130:898-902.

27. Dorairajan LN, Gupta H, Kumar S. Pelvic fracture–associated urethral injuries in girls: experience with primary repair. BJU Int 2004;94:134-6.

28. Elliott DS, Barrett DM. Long-term follow up and evaluation of primary realignment of posterior urethral disruptions. J Urol 1997;157:814-6.

29. Turner-Warwick R. Prevention of complications resulting from pelvic fracture urethral injuries— and from their surgical management. Urol Clin North Am 1989;16:335-58.

30. Routt ML, Simonian PT, Defalco AJ, et al. Internal fixation in pelvic fractures and primary repairs of associated genitourinary disruptions: a team approach. J Trauma 1996;40:784-90.

31. Flynn BJ, Delvecchio FC, Webster GD. Perineal repair of pelvic fracture urethral distraction defects: experience in 120 patients during the last 10 years. J Urol 2003;170:1877–80.

32. Koraitim MM. On the art of anastomotic posterior urethroplasty: a 27-year experience. J Urol 2005;173:135–9.

33. Kamdar C, Mooppan UM, Kim H, et al. Penile fracture: preoperative evaluation and surgical technique for optimal patient outcome. BJU008;102:1640–4.

34. Brock G, Hsu G, Nunes L, et al. The anatomy of the tunica albuginea in the normal penis and Peyronie's disease. J Urol 1997;157:276–81.

35. Mazaris EM, Livadas K, Chalikopoulos D, et al. Penile fractures: immediate surgical approach with a midline ventral incision. BJU Int 2009;104:520–3.

36. Kanegaye JT, Schonfeld N. Penile zipper entrapment: a simple and less threatening approach using mineral oil. Pediatr Emerg Care 1993;9:90–1.

37. Oosterlinck W. Unbloody management of penile zipper injury. Eur Urol 1981;7:365–6.

38. Saraf P, Rabinowitz R. Zipper injury of the foreskin. Am J Dis Child 1982;136:557–8.

Chapter 19

GYNAECOLOGIC EMERGEMCIES

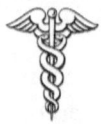

Vandana Jain

Acute gynecological emergencies are a common cause of morbidity and mortality among women of reproductive age group worldwide.

Gynecological emergencies visits account for 24.3 visits per thousand women of reproductive age group (15–44 years) in developed world.[1]

Although similar data for developing countries is not readily available, it presents enormous challenges on the weak healthcare infrastructure of such countries.

Gynecological emergencies can be broadly classified into pregnancy related and non-pregnancy related emergencies.

Pregnancy related emergencies include complications of early pregnancy like ectopic pregnancy, miscarriage and unsafe abortion.

Non-pregnancy related complications include pelvic inflammatory disease (PID), complications related to ovarian cysts, menstrual disorders, bleeding of gynecological malignancies, coital lacerations and sexual assault.

1. ECTOPIC PREGNANCY

Tubal ectopic pregnancy is the most common of all types of ectopic pregnancies and will be discussed in this article. The most common etiological factor is salpingitis.[2] Other causes include hormonal disturbances, smoking, altered tubal anatomy and tubo-ovarian relationship due to pelvic masses or pelvic adhesions.

CLINICAL FEATURES

The most common presenting symptoms are abdominal pain, amenorrhea and vaginal bleeding and can be associated with history of dizziness or fainting. The most common signs are abdominal tenderness, adnexal tenderness or an adnexal mass. Signs of peritoneal irritation might be present in patients with Hemoperitoneum.

WORKUP & INVESTIGATIONS

Transvaginal ultrasound (TVS) is the gold standard for diagnosis of tubal ectopic pregnancy and usually visualizes an adnexal mass that moves separate to the ovary. In the absence of adnexal mass, it can be diagnosed if an intrauterine gestational sac is absent, while the serum β-HCG levels are above the discriminatory zone (β-HCG levels between 1500–2000 mIU/ml for TVS) with good accuracy.[3] Furthermore, if the β-HCG levels are below the discriminatory zone and patient is stable clinically, then serial β-HCG levels can be done. About 85% of normal intrauterine conceptions have an increase of 66% or more in β-HCG levels in 48 hours as compared to only 13% of ectopic pregnancies demonstrating this 66% rise.[4]

Sometimes, it is important to differentiate an ectopic pregnancy from inevitable abortion. This can be done by performing a dilatation and curettage, once an abnormal gestation is confirmed by abnormal β-HCG levels, and sending the tissue to pathology department. Presence of chorionic villi rules out an ectopic pregnancy, unless it is a case of heterotopic pregnancy. A repeat β-HCG level 24 hour after a dilatation and curettage should fall by about 50%.

MANAGEMENT

Expectant Management

- Absence of pain

- Hemodynamically stable

- Unruptured tubal mass < 35 mm with no fetal cardiac activity

- Adequately counselled woman willing for follow up

- Serum β-HCG levels less than 1000 mIU/ml

Medical Management

Methotrexate is the most commonly used drug. Methotrexate is given under medical surveillance, after hospitalizing the patient and a viable intrauterine pregnancy must be completely ruled out before giving methotrexate.

Indications

- Hemodynamic stability

- Unruptured ectopic pregnancy with tubal mass < 35 mm, with no fetal cardiac activity

- Certainty of absence of intrauterine gestation

- Low serum β-HCG levels, ideally less than 1500 mIU/ml but can be up to 5000 mIU/ml

- No known sensitivity or contraindications to methotrexate

Contraindications

- Pre-existing blood dyscrasia

- Abnormal renal function

- Hepatic Dysfunction

- Active pulmonary disease

- Peptic ulcer disease

- Breastfeeding

Protocol

Single dose regimen with intramuscular dose of 50 mg/m^2 is preferred over the multiple dose regimen. CBC,

LFT, KFT, Blood group and serum β-HCG levels are done on day of injection (Day 1) and serum β-HCG level is repeated on Day 4 and 7. A fall of 15% or more in β-HCG levels between Day 4 and 7 is considered as satisfactory and β-HCG levels should be repeated weekly till levels fall below 15 mIU/ml. If the fall in β-HCG levels is less than 15% as occurs in about 20% women, then a second dose of methotrexate can be given after excluding ectopic fetal cardiac activity and presence of haemoperitoneum by a repeat transvaginal ultrasound.[5] Highest success rates (90%) are seen with initial β-HCG levels are less than 5000 mIU/ml.

However, patient may require surgery if the serum β-HCG rises and patient develops signs and symptoms suggestive of ruptured ectopic pregnancy. Patient should not take alcohol and folate containing vitamins during treatment.

Surgical Management

Majority of tubal ectopic pregnancies are managed surgically. Laparoscopic salpingotomy

Or salpingectomy is preferred over laparotomy unless the patient is hemodynamically unstable or the required expertise and equipment for laparoscopic surgery is not available.

Laparoscopy is associated with shorter operating time, lesser chances of adhesion formation, and faster recovery and shorter length of hospital stay.[6]

Salpingotomy is associate with greater risk of persistent trophoblastic disease compared to laparotomy (7% versus less than 1%).[7] Repeat β-HCG levels are recommended 7 days after salpingotomy and weekly thereafter till a negative result is obtained.

Also, the chances of repeat ectopic pregnancy are 8% with salpingotomy compared to 5% with salpingectomy.[7] Moreover, the cumulative pregnancy rates have found to been found to be equivalent with salpingotomy and salpingectomy in presence of healthy contralateral tube.

Thus, RGOC guidelines recommend that salpingectomy should be performed in preference to salpingotomy in patients with healthy contralateral tube.

Salpingotomy should be performed in women with damaged contralateral tube or a history of fertility reducing factors like previous ectopic pregnancy, previous abdominal surgery or a history of PID.[8] However, they must be explained that they might require methotrexate or salpingectomy if there is persistent trophoblastic disease or bleeding.

I. COMPLICATIONS OF UNSAFE ABORTION

Unsafe abortion is defined by the WHO as the termination of an unintended pregnancy either by persons lacking the necessary skills or in an environment lacking the minimal medical standards, or both.[9]

Methods of unsafe abortion include oral intake of toxic fluids, inflicting direct injury to cervix, vagina or uterus by inserting herbal preparations or foreign bodies or inflicting external trauma to abdomen and performing improper dilatation and curettage by unskilled providers under unhygienic conditions.

Despite liberalization of abortion laws in a number of developing countries, unsafe abortion still persists as a public health concern. About 90% of unsafe abortions occur in developing countries where a large proportion of women do not have access to safe abortion services due to combination of social, economic, religious and legal factors.[10] Complications of unsafe abortions are a leading cause of morbidity and mortality in developing countries, mostly due to hemorrhaged, disseminated intravascular coagulopathy (DIC), sepsis, peritonitis, renal failure, chemical burns or drug toxicity and trauma to genital tract and abdominal viscera.

Factors responsible for increased morbidity and mortality associated with unsafe abortions:

- Lack of provider skill
- Poor technique
- Unsanitary conditions
- Lack of appropriate equipment
- Use of toxic substances
- Poor maternal health
- Increased gestational age
- Lack of access to post abortion cares services

Management of Complications

When a woman in reproductive age group presents with conditions related to genital tract, pregnancy should always be kept in mind. A thorough history should be taken including a history of recent abortion, exposure to chemicals, ingestion of toxic substances or instrumentation. Unsafe abortion must be considered a possibility even in countries where the process of abortion is legal.

Clinical examination includes assessment of vital signs, vaginal bleeding, trauma to genital tract, and whether signs of uterine infection like fever, tachycardia, foul smelling vaginal discharge or uterine tenderness are present.

After initial resuscitation with I/V fluids, broad spectrum antibiotics, painkillers and control of uterine bleeding with uterine massage, uterotonic agents or vaginal/intrauterine pack, patients with heavy bleeding, abdominal pain, and those with features of infection or shock should be transported to centers with availability of blood transfusion facilities and surgical expertise.

If the uterus is atonic, uterine massage should be done along with administration of uterotonic agents (misoprostol 800 mcg per rectally or methylergonovine 0.2 mg orally or intramuscularly). It is important to rule out retained products of conception, especially if there is no response to uterotonic agents, and the uterus should be evacuated using suction evacuation or dilatation and curettage under antibiotic coverage. In unresponsive cases, tamponade with intrauterine pack or balloon may be effective in controlling uterine atony.

Traumatic injuries to the genital tract are usually the culprit in patients bleeding profusely despite the presence of normal uterine tone. Actively bleeding lower genital tract lacerations must be repair surgically, usually in an operation theatre, with proper exposure and asepsis. Exploratory laparotomy is usually needed in patients with extensive lacerations extending into the abdominal cavity and in those with trauma to abdominal viscera and blood vessels.

Preventive Measures

Strategies are required at three different levels to reduce the frequency and severity of complications associated with unsafe abortion.[11] ***Primary prevention*** includes easy access to contraceptives, legalization of abortion on request and improving the skills of the service providers. WHO recommends manual vacuum aspiration as the preferred method for uterine evacuation before 12 weeks of gestation, and combined use of mifepristone and misoprostol as the standard regimen for early medical termination of pregnancy.[12] ***Secondary prevention*** includes prompt evacuation of the products of conception from the uterine cavity in case of incomplete abortion by either misoprostol or by manual vacuum aspiration along with prompt empirical antibiotic therapy to prevent the infections and the resulting morbidity. ***Tertiary prevention*** involves management of life threatening complications like perforated uterus with gut prolapse or repair of bowel and bladder fistula.

In addition to provision of safe abortion services, need of post abortion care needs to be emphasized. Post abortion care includes management of complications of incomplete abortion like bleeding, sepsis or genital tract injuries, provision of family planning services and counselling so that unintended pregnancies can be avoided, and referral for other reproductive health care needs.

II. PELVIC INFLAMMATORY DISEASE

Pelvic inflammatory disease (PID) comprises a spectrum of inflammatory disorders of upper female genital tract, including any combination of endometritis, salpingitis, Tubo-ovarian abscess and pelvic peritonitis.[13]

Acute PID is the most common Non- pregnancy related gynaecological emergency.

Most common organisms implicated in the pathogenesis are N. gonorrhoeae and C. trachomatis, others being anaerobes, G. vaginalis, H. influenza, S. agalactie, CMV, M. hominis, U. urealyticus and M. genitalium.[14-16]

Diagnosis of PID may be difficult due to wide variations in the signs and symptoms. Many episodes of PID may go unrecognized. Sometimes the healthcare provider may fail to recognize mild symptoms and signs like bleeding, dyspareunia and vaginal discharge.

Delay in diagnosis might predispose the affected women to future risk of infertility, ectopic pregnancy and chronic pelvic pain.

CDC Criteria for Diagnosis of PID

Minimum Criteria

- Cervical motion tenderness
- Uterine tenderness
- Adnexal tenderness

Additional Criteria

- Oral temperature > 101°F (> 38.3°C)

- Abnormal cervical mucopurulent discharge or cervical fragility

- Presence of abundant number of WBCs on saline microscopy of vaginal fluid

- Elevated ESR

- Elevated C Reactive protein

- Documented cervical infection with N. Gonorrhoeae or C. Trachomatis

Presence of one or more additional criteria in addition to one of three minimal criteria increases the specificity of diagnosis of PID.

The most specific criteria for diagnosis of PID include:

- Endometrial biopsy with histopathological evidence of endometritis

- TVS or MRI showing thick fluid filled tubes with or without free pelvic fluid or Tubo-ovarian abscess or Doppler studies suggesting pelvic infection.

- Laparoscopic findings consistent with PID

Empirical treatment with broad spectrum antibiotics should be started as soon as the presumptive diagnosis of PID is made to prevent the long-term sequel. Combination of antibiotics should be used due to polymicrobial nature of the disease.

Any regimen used to treat PID should be effective against N. Gonorrhoeae and C. Trachomatis and facultative aerobes and anaerobes, particularly those associated with bacterial vaginosis.

Patients with mild to moderately severe PID can be managed as outpatients with intramuscular/oral therapy. Women who do not respond within 72 hours should be admitted, reevaluated for diagnosis, and administered intravenous therapy.

Recommended I/M or oral regimens:

1. Ceftriaxone 250 mg I/M single dose

   PLUS

   Doxycycline 100 mg orally twice a day x 14 days

      WITH or WITHOUT

      Metronidazole 500 mg twice a day x 14 days

2. Cefoxitin 2 gm I/M single dose and Probenecid 1 gm orally concurrently in a single dose

   PLUS

   Doxycycline 100 mg twice a day x 14 days

      WITH or WITHOUT

      Metronidazole 500 mg twice a day x 14 days

3. Other parenteral third generation cephalosporin (like ceftizoxime or cefotaxime)

   PLUS

   Doxycycline 100 mg twice daily x 14 days

      WITH or WITHOUT

      Metronidazole 500 mg twice daily x 14 days

Indications of Hospitalization

- Uncertain diagnosis and surgical emergencies (e.g. appendicitis) cannot be ruled out

- Pregnancy

- Severe illness, nausea and vomiting, high fever

- Patient is unable to follow or tolerate outpatient treatment

- No clinical response to oral antimicrobial therapy

- Presence of tubo-ovarian abscess

Recommended parenteral treatment regimens:

1. Cefotetan 2 gm I/V every 12 hours

   PLUS

   Doxycycline 100 mg orally or I/V every 12 hours

2. Cefoxitin 2 gm I/V every 6 hours

   PLUS

   Doxycycline 100 mg orally or I/V every 12 hours

3. Clindamycin 900 mg I/V every 8 hours

   PLUS

   Gentamycin loading dose I/V or I/M (2 mg/kg) followed by maintenance dose 1.5 mg/kg every 8 hours

When using parenteral Cefotetan and Cefoxitin based regimens, oral treatment with doxycycline 100 mg twice daily can be initiated 48 hours after clinical improvement to complete the 14 days of treatment.

For Clindamycin/Gentamycin regimens, oral treatment with clindamycin 450 mg 4 times a day or doxycycline 100 mg twice daily can be used to complete the 14 days of treatment.

Special Circumstances

- **Tubo-Ovarian Abscess**

  ➤ All patients with Tubo-ovarian abscess must be hospitalized and parenteral treatment should be started with clindamycin and gentamycin.

  ➤ If no improvement occurs in 48 hours, then one can consider drainage of the abscess. The abscess fluid should be sent for culture and sensitivity and the drain should be left behind for 48 hours.

  ➤ Surgery with emergency laparotomy is usually needed in patients with ruptured Tubo - ovarian masses and in those with persistent tubo- ovarian masses despite parenteral antibiotics, who no longer desire fertility

- **Adolescents and HIV positive patients** can be managed with same outpatient regimens as others and there is insufficient evidence that they require more aggressive management like hospitalization or parenteral I/V regimens

- **IUCD users** need not get the IUCD removed on diagnosis of PID. However, if no clinical improvement to treatment occurs in 48–72 hours then the health care provider can consider removing the IUCD.

Follow Up

Sexual partners of the patient should be traced and adequately treated and patient should refrain from sexual activity till the therapy is completed.

All women diagnosed and treated for chlamydial or gonococcal PID should be retested 3 months after treatment.

III. EMERGENCIES ASSOCIATED WITH ADENEXAL MASSES

- TORSION
- RUPTURE
- HAEMORRHAGE
- INFECTION

Torsion

The most common etiological factor associated with torsion is presence of an adnexal mass, usually the ones with size ranging from 8 to 12 cm.[17] The most common ovarian tumor to undergo torsion is dermoid cyst due to its characteristic size and density.

Other conditions which increase the risk of torsion are hyperstimulated ovaries associated with in vitro fertilization, and pregnancy, where, as the uterus enlarges and comes out of pelvis, it pushes the ovaries anteriorly causing torsion.

Rupture

Rupture of an ovarian cyst can occur spontaneously or may be triggered by abdominal trauma. Rupture of a small cyst may go unnoticed but rupture of a large cyst, especially with irritant contents like dermoid cyst/endometriotic cyst can cause symptoms of peritonitis.

Hemorrhage

Small hemorrhages can occur in normal ovulatory ovaries leading to formation of corpus luteal cyst.

Hemorrhage can occur from the edge of ruptured ovarian cyst or a ruptured corpus luteal cyst and can lead to intraperitoneal bleed, especially if the patient has some underlying bleeding disorder or if the patient is on anticoagulant therapy.

Infection

Tubo-ovarian abscess can form in patients with PID. Endometriotic cysts and dermoid cysts can also become infected. Rupture of an infected cyst can lead to peritonitis.

Clinical Features

All of the abovementioned conditions are associated with symptoms of acute abdomen. Torsion of an adnexal mass usually present as acute or subacute intermittent pelvic pain associated with nausea, vomiting and mild fever. Examination usually reveals tenderness in lower abdomen and a tender adnexal mass may be felt on per-vaginal examination.

Patients with hemorrhagic ovarian cyst may present with hypovolemia and hemodynamic instability. Tubo-ovarian abscess can present with symptoms of PID like discharge per vaginum, fever and Abdomino-pelvic pain and tender pelvic masses on examination.

Workup & Investigations

Conditions like ectopic pregnancy, appendicitis, urinary tract infections, renal colic, bowel obstruction, mesenteric ischemia, acute diverticulitis and acute PID can mimic the above-mentioned conditions and they should be excluded by taking detailed history, thorough physical examination and relevant investigations. Simple investigations like urine for pregnancy test can rule out ectopic pregnancy. A complete blood count might reveal low Hemoglobin in hemorrhagic ovarian cyst or a low platelet count in patients with bleeding disorders. Leukocytosis might be evident in patients with torsion or tubo-ovarian abscess.

Cervical swabs for chlamydia and gonorrhea can help in diagnosing PID.

A simple imaging modality like ultrasound might reveal the characteristic features of dermoid cyst or endometriotic cyst. Free fluid with internal echoes might suggest an intraperitoneal bleed or cyst fluid in hemorrhagic or ruptured ovarian cyst. Color Doppler flow study along with pelvic ultrasound can be very useful in diagnosing adnexal torsion with high accuracy.[18] Sometimes a CT scan might be required to rule out appendicitis and other surgical emergencies.

Management

A small hemorrhagic cyst with mild symptoms can be managed conservatively and followed up after 4 to 6 weeks with a repeat ultrasound. Oral contraceptive medication may also be given for 3 to 6 cycles if the cyst is not increasing in size.

Most of the complicated ovarian cysts will require surgical intervention which can be laparoscopic or a laparotomy depending upon the clinical scenario.

Depending upon the situation an ovarian cystectomy or salpingo-oopherectomy may be required. If the adenexal mass appears suspicious for malignancy it is better to convert to laparotomy to avoid any rupture or spillage and perform a salpingo-oopherectomy.

Most of the cases of adenexal torsion can be managed laparoscopically and a gentle untwisting of ovarian pedicle followed by Oophoropexy to pelvic side wall can be done.[19] However, once severe vascular compromise sets in and the ovarian tissue becomes completely infarcted and necrotic, salpingo-oopherectomy remains the only viable option to resort to.

Care must be taken during salpingo-oopherectomy for adenexal torsion as the ureter is usually lifted up and can be injured while clamping the infundibulopelvic ligament.

IV. GYNECOLOGIC HEMORRHAGE

Gynecologic hemorrhage can be classified into abnormal uterine bleeding (AUB), when there is an organic cause for it, either systemic or local, or dysfunctional uterine bleeding (DUB), when no organic cause can be found.

Systemic organic causes include bleeding disorders, chronic liver disease, chronic kidney disease, hypothyroidism etc. Local causes include various complications of early pregnancy, genital tract malignancies, fibroids, infection, trauma and foreign bodies.

Dysfunctional bleeding can be further classified into anovulatory uterine bleeding and ovulatory uterine bleeding.

Abnormal and excessive uterine bleeding can manifest as menorrhagia or metrorrhagia.

Menorrhagia is defined as menstrual cycles occurring at regular intervals ranging from 21 to 35 days, but the blood flow lasts for more than 7 days or the amount of blood loss is more than 80 ml.

Metrorrhagia is defined as excessive and frequent menstruation with irregular cycles.

Clinical Features

Patients may present with symptoms of anemia like fatigue, lethargy or breathlessness. On general examination, pallor, pedal edema and tachycardia may be present and on gynecological examination, findings suggestive of reproductive tract pathology like, discharge, cervical lesion, enlarged uterus or adnexal mass may be evident.

Workup & Investigations

To evaluate the cause of abnormal bleeding, basic investigations like a complete blood count, coagulation profile, liver function test, kidney function test and a thyroid function test should be ordered. A pregnancy test must be done to rule out pregnancy. An ultrasound scan can detect coarse hepatic architecture in patients with chronic liver disease and reproductive tract abnormalities like elevated endometrial thickness, uterine polyp or growth, fibroids, tubo-ovarian masses or cervical lesions.

A Pap's smear should be taken if the cervix is suspicious and a cervical biopsy should be taken if there is an obvious cervical growth.

Patients at risk of endometrial cancer, like patients older that 35 years of age, those with history of unopposed estrogen usage, obesity or chronic anovulation and those with postmenopausal bleeding should be evaluated with an office endometrial biopsy. In patients with inadequate tissue on pipelle biopsy, a diagnostic hysteroscopy and endometrial biopsy should be planned.

Management

After initial stabilization of clinically unstable patients with intravascular fluid therapy and transfusion of blood products further treatment should only be initiated after the etiology of AUB has been evaluated and premalignant and malignant disease process has been excluded. The goal of therapy is to control the bleeding, treat anemia and treat the underlying cause.

Patients with endocrine and infectious disorders should be treated medically (e.g., polycystic ovarian syndrome or chronic endometritis). Patients with hypothyroidism respond to treatment with L- thyroxine. Patients with chronic liver disease should be evaluated in collaboration with gastroenterologist. AUB associated with structural lesions in the uterine cavity like endometrial polyp and submucosal fibroid should be managed with hysteroscopic resection. Patients with incomplete or missed abortion should be managed with dilatation and curettage, while patients with threatened abortion can be managed with bed rest and evaluations with serial serum β-HCG and transvaginal ultrasound.

Adolescent patients with abnormal uterine bleeding can have an underlying coagulopathy or bleeding disorder in about 20% cases and need to be treated accordingly if any disorder is detected.[20] In patients with Von Willebrand disease, the mainstay of treatment is DDAVP (desmopressin acetate) which comes in form of injection and as nasal spray. Recombinant VWF is used to treat patients with severe forms of VWD or those who do not respond to desmopressin nasal spray. Antifibrinolytic agents like tranexamic acid can be given orally or by intravenous route to prevent the breakdown of clots. In patients who do not respond to these initial measures might require an examination under anesthesia or a dilatation and curettage.[21]

The initial approach to control acute menorrhagia, particularly when the bleeding has been prolonged or very heavy is to administer high dose conjugated estrogen to stabilize the endometrium. Premarin can be given in a dose of 25 mg intravenous every 4 hours till bleeding stops. Patients who require high doses of conjugated estrogen will also require high doses of progestin (norethindrone acetate 5 mg 4 times a day) to counteract the estrogenic effects. Patient usually responds in 6 to 12 hours to hormonal therapy. Alternatively, oral contraceptive pill (OCP) containing 35–50 mcg of Ethinyl estradiol can be given three times a day for 3 days followed by twice a day for 3 days followed by once daily till the pack is finished. Patient should be provided with antiemetic drugs and should be given leg stockings or other intermittent self-compression devices as use of high dose estrogen therapy is associated with nausea and increased risk of thrombotic events. Cyclical combined oral contraceptive pills or cyclic oral progestin therapy (e.g., oral medroxy-progesterone acetate, 10 mg tablet daily for 10–14 days) can also be used in anovulatory dysfunctional bleeding once acute bleeding episode has been controlled.[22] Tranexamic acid or nonsteroidal anti-inflammatory drugs (NSAIDs) are useful for patients with heavy menstrual bleeding who have contraindications to or would prefer to avoid hormonal agents.

Patients with operable gynecologic malignancies like endometrial cancer or early stage cervical cancer should undergo surgery after proper evaluation. Patients with locally advanced cervical or vaginal cancers who present with severe acute hemorrhage can be managed by vaginal packing and blood transfusion. Haemostatic dose of external beam radiation might me required for cases not responding to vaginal packing.

V. INJURIES TO GENITAL STRUCTURES

Vaginal bleeding, vaginal lacerations, anal tears and rectal injuries can occur during rough and hurried coitus due to inexperience or rape. Sometimes the perpetrators deliberately introduce sharp objects into the vagina of the victims leading to fistula formation, gut prolapse, injury to bowel, bladder or other pelvic viscera.

Vulvar and vaginal hematomas can occur secondary to blunt trauma like saddle injuries, automobile accidents, recreational activities or due to spontaneous rupture of varicosities in peripartum period.

Vulvar hematoma presents as painful mass in the labial region, while a vaginal hematoma though associated with symptoms like difficulty in voiding or defecating, might only be identified after an internal examination.

Victims of sexual assault or rape require detailed history and physical examination. It usually requires the involvement of police and forensic experts.

Management

Management of genital injuries involves resuscitation of patients with intravenous fluids and blood products and exploration and repair of vaginal or anal lacerations in operation theatre. Broad spectrum antibiotics should be started in all cases. Emergency laparotomy might be required in patients with haemoperitoneum, retroperitoneal hematomas, deep vaginal lacerations extending through pouch of Douglas into the peritoneal cavity and in patients with pelvic visceral injuries. A diverting colostomy might be required in patients with deep anal lacerations, requiring involvement of a general surgeon. Victims of sexual assault should be provided with post-exposure prophylaxis for HIV depending upon the risk, tested to exclude pregnancy and should be provided with emergency contraception and prophylactically vaccinated against hepatitis B.

For patients with history of blunt trauma, especially road traffic accidents, pelvic fractures and injuries to bowel, bladder and peritoneal cavity should be ruled out. Some form of anesthesia, topical, intravenous or regional, may be required before examination of such patients.

A Foley catheter should be placed as urinary retention can occur with expanding hematomas.

Radiographic evaluation might be required if internal injuries are suspected.

Management of vulvar or vaginal hematomas is usually conservative. Most hematomas are venous in nature, are self-limiting and respond to ice packs and compression. Arterial hematomas are usually rapidly expanding and require exploration, identification and ligation of the bleeding vessel. If the bleeding site cannot be identified, internal iliac or uterine artery embolization can be performed.[23]

Follow Up

Patients should be prescribed Sitz baths two to three times a day until the lacerations heal. Pelvic rest is also recommended for three to four weeks to prevent disruption of healing tissue. Appropriate analgesics, anti-inflammatory agents and antibiotics should be prescribed. Patient counselling and psychological support should be an integral part of follow up as women who suffer trauma of the genital tract are more likely to experience dyspareunia, sexual dysfunction and chronic pelvic pain in future.[24]

Conclusions

Gynecological emergencies are a common cause of morbidity and mortality, especially in developing countries. Most of the emergencies have signs and symptoms which overlap with common surgical causes like acute appendicitis, acute diverticulitis, ureteric colic etc. which need to be excluded by appropriate examination and investigations.

Timely and diligent management of most of the gynecological emergencies can prevent catastrophic consequences, allowing the overburdened healthcare systems a sigh of relief.

REFERENCES

1. Curtis KM, Hillis SD, Kieke BA, et al. Visits to emergency departments for gynecologic disorders in the United States, 1992-1994. Obstet Gynecol 1998; 91: 1007-1012.

2. Westrom L, Bengtsson LP, Mardh PA. Incidence, trends, and risks of ectopic pregnancy in a population of women. Br med J (Clin Res Ed) 1981; 282: 15-8.

3. Varma R, Mascarenhas L. Evidence-based management of ectopic pregnancy. Curr Obstet Gynecol 2002; 12: 191-199.

4. Kadar N, Caldwell BV, Romero R. A method of screening for ectopic pregnancy and its indications. Obstet Gynecol 1981; 58: 162-166.

5. Stovall TG, Ling FW, Gray LA. Single-dose methotrexate for treatment of ectopic pregnancy. Obstet Gynecol 1991; 77: 754-757.

6. Lundorff P, Thorburn J, Hahlin M, et al. Laparoscopic surgery in ectopic pregnancy. A randomized trial versus laparotomy. Acta Obstet Gynecol Scand 1991; 70: 343-348.

7. Mol F, van Mello NM, Strandell K, et al. European surgery in ectopic pregnancy (ESEP) study group. Salpingotomy versus salpingectomy in women with tubal pregnancy (ESEP study): an open-label, multicenter, randomised controlled trial. Lancet 2014; 383: 1483-1489.

8. Becker S, Solomayer E, Hornung R, et al. Optimal treatment for patients with ectopic pregnancies and a history of fertility-reducing factors. Arch Gynecol Obstet 2011; 283: 41-45.

9. World Health Organization. Unsafe abortion, authors. Global and Regional Estimates of the Incidence of Unsafe Abortion and Associated Mortality in 2003. 5th ed. Geneva: World Health Organization; 2007.

10. Singh S. The incidence of unsafe abortion: A global review. In: Warriner IK, Shah IH, eds., Preventing unsafe abortion and its consequences: Priorities for research and action, New York: Guttmacher Institute, 2006.

11. Grimes DA, Benson J, Singh S, et al. Unsafe abortion: the preventable pandemic. Lancet 2006; 368: 1908-1919.

12. World Health Organization. Safe abortion: technical and policy guidance for health systems. Geneva: World Health Organization, 2003.

13. Wiesenfeld HC, Sweet RL, Ness RB, et al. Comparison of acute and subclinical pelvic inflammatory disease. Sex Transm Dis 2005; 32: 400-405.

14. Burnett AM, Anderson CP, Zwank MD. Laboratory-confirmed gonorrhea and/or chlamydia rates in clinically diagnosed pelvic inflammatory disease and cervicitis. Am J Emerg Med 2012; 30: 1114–1117.

15. Ness RB, Kip KE, Hillier SL, et al. A cluster analysis of bacterial vaginosis-associated microflora and pelvic inflammatory disease. Am J Epidemiol 2005; 162: 585–590.

16. Haggerty CL, Totten PA, Astete SG, et al. *Mycoplasma genitalium* among women with nongonococcal, nonchlamydial pelvic inflammatory disease. Infect Dis Obstet Gynecol 2006:30184.

17. Stenchever MA, Droegemueller W, Herbst AL, et al. Comprehensive gynecology. 4th edition. Philadelphia: Mosby; 2001. P. 519

18. Albayam F, Hamper UM. Ovarian and adnexal torsion: spectrum of sonographic findings with pathologic correlation. J Ultrasound Med 2001; 20: 1083-1089.

19. Cohen SB, Wattiez A, Seidman DS, et al. Laparoscopy versus laparotomy for detorsion and sparing of twisted ischemic adnexa. JSLS 2003; 7: 295-299.

20. Claessens EA, Cowell CA. Acute adolescent menorrhagia. Am J Obstet Gynecol 1981; 139: 277-280.

21. Screening and management of bleeding disorders in adolescents with heavy menstrual bleeding: ACOG COMMITTEE OPINION, Number 785. Obstet Gynecol 2019; 134: e71-e83.

22. Chuong CJ, Brenner PF. Management of abnormal uterine bleeding. Am J Obstet Gynecol 1996; 175: 787-792.

23. Kunishima K, Takao H, Kato N, et al. Transarterial embolization of a nonpuerperal traumatic vulvar hematoma. Radiat Med 2008; 26: 168-170.

24. Harlow BL, Wise LA, Stewart EG. Prevalence and predictors of chronic lower genital tract discomfort. Am J Obstet Gynecol 2001; 185: 545-550.

Chapter 20

NANOTECHNOLOGY AND THE SURGEON

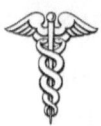

Sonia

Surgery involves an early diagnosis, followed by surgery and postoperative care.

For proper treatment, diagnostic modalities should be perfect for successful surgery. Nanotechnology is used in MRI, ultrasound and nuclear imaging modalities. Surgeons are interested in minimally invasive methods to treat their patients. Scalpel and needles are affected by nanotechnology. Thus with the use of nano-technology, there is minimum trauma during surgery and minimum postoperative complications.

Nanotechnology can be used to synthesize tiny biosensors which can shorten a patient's recovery period and save on hospital stay.

WOUND DRESSINGS

Metallic silver is known for its anti-infective properties, which are effective against a wide range of bacteria and microorganisms. A nano-porous silver powder, which can be applied to a range of products, has been developed. Smaller particles give a greater surface area, and, therefore, a better anti-infective surface. Also, less silver is required overall, so there is less risk of any toxic side effects.

Applications for nano-silver coatings on medical devices include implants, indwelling catheters and wound dressings, and for burns and other chronic wounds.

NANOROBOTS

Nanotechnology is used to produce nanorobots or nanobots. These miniature robots are so small that they can be introduced into the body either through the vascular system or through catheters, and with external guidance and monitoring by the surgeon they can perform precise intracellular surgery, which would not be possible with the human hand.

TISSUE ENGINEERING

Tissue engineering has been defined as 'the application of principles and methods of engineering and life sciences towards fundamental understanding of structure-function relationships in normal and pathological mammalian tissues and thus to improve tissue function'. Tissue-engineered products typically are a combination of three components, i.e. isolated cells, an extracellular matrix and signal molecules, such as growth factors.

CATHETER FOR MINIMALLY INVASIVE SURGERY

Catheters are small tubes which are inserted into the body cavity to inject or drain fluids or to keep a passageway clear. As catheters are foreign bodies, there is a chance of thrombus formation on the surface of these devices. Nanomaterials, e.g. carbon nanotubes, have been successfully added to catheters used in minimally invasive surgery to increase their strength and flexibility and reduce their thrombogenic effect.

NANOCOATED SURGICAL BLADE

The performance of surgical blades has been enhanced significantly by coating surgical blades with diamond with the help of nanotechnology. Major advantages of the diamond nanolayers in this application are low physical adhesion to materials or tissues and chemical/biological inertness. In addition, diamond has a low friction coefficient, decreasing the penetration force necessary. Advances in novel manufacturing methods have enabled the production of surgical blades with a cutting edge diameter in the region of 5 nm–1 μm. The diamond scalpels with a cutting edge of only a few atoms (approximately 3 nm) have been made for applications in eye, neurosurgery and minimal invasive surgery. The width of the scalpel blade is approximately one thousandth of a metal blade.

NANONEEDLES

New suture needles for ophthalmic and plastic surgery are made of stainless steel, incorporating nano-sized particles (1–10 nm quasicrystals) by using thermal ageing techniques. Such needles have good ductility, exceptional strength and corrosion resistance. The sizes of these nanoneedles are 200–300 nm in diameter, and 6–8 μm in length. By modifying the surface of a nanoneedle, various molecules such as DNA, proteins or chemicals can be loaded using standard immobilization techniques.

FEMTOSECOND LASER

A femtosecond laser is a laser which emits ultrashort optical pulses with durations in the range of femtoseconds (1 fs = 10–15 s). These lasers belong to the category of ultrafast lasers or ultrashort pulse lasers capable of creating intensities in the range of $10^{13/cm2}$. Their ease of use, precision, and ability to localize light, make them excellent tools for the manipulation of structures and biological molecules. Femtosecond lasers have been used to cut and reshape the cornea to correct vision in humans. Using a femtosecond laser, the damage caused to the endothelial tissues on the surface of the cornea has been eliminated. These lasers have also been used to cut single acting stress fibers in living cells and study the changes in cell shape, and to cut chromosomes. They have also been used to remove mitochondria from living cells while retaining cell division. This demonstrates the use of lasers for nano-surgery to remove specific organelles without affecting long-term viability.

Progressions in nanobiotechnology are transforming our capability to understand biological intricacies and resolve biological and medical problems by developing subtle biomimetic techniques. Preliminary investigations support the potential of nano-biomaterials in orthopaedic applications; however, significant advancements are necessary to achieve clinical use. The research areas of implanted interfaces, tissue engineering and therapeutics have been in focus over many years.. Nanotechnology has made the surgeons' life easier by use of surgical tools such as nanoneedles, nano-surgical blades, better diagnostic imaging and better postoperative treatment, by using precisely targeted delivery systems for the medicine.

REFERENCE

1. Bogedal M, Glieche M, Geibert JC, Hoffschulz H, Laccateli S, Malsh I, et al. Nanotechnology and its implications for the health of the EU citizen, www.nanoforum.org. Link checked 3/10/201

2. Freitas RA. What is nanomedicine? Nanomed Nanotechnol Biol Med. 2005;1:2e9. doi: 10.1016/j.nano.2004.11.003. [CrossRef] [Google Scholar]

3. Freitas RA (2005) Nanotechnology, nanomedicine and nanosurgery. Int J Surg 3(4):243–246 [PubMed]

4. Abhilash M. Nanorobots. Int J Pharma Bio Sci. 2010;1(1):1–10. [Google Scholar]

5. Roszek B, de Jong WH, Geertsma RE, Nanotechnology in medical applications: state-

of-the-art in materials and devices, RIVM report. 265001001,

6. Implants, Surgery and Coatings. http://www. observatorynano.eu/project/filesystem/files/ Surgery,%20implants%20and%20coatings-April%2009.pdf

7. Mritunjai S, et al. Nanotechnology in medicine and antibacterial effect of silver nanoparticles. Digest J Nanomater Biostruct. 2008;3(3):115–122. [Google Scholar]

8. Tareen T. Nanotechnology in Medicine, www. medlink-uk.org/Site/documents/Nano2011/.pdf. Link checked 3/10/2011

9. Juhasz T, Loesel FH, Kurtz RM, Horvath C, Bille JF, Mourou G. Corneal refractive surgery with femtosecond lasers. IEEE J Sel Top Quantum Electron. 1999;5:902–910. doi: 10.1109/2944.796309. [CrossRef] [Google Scholar]

10. Yanik MF, Cinar H, Cinar HN, Chisholm AD, Jin Y, Ben Yakar A. Neurosurgery: Functional regeneration after laser axotomy. Nature. 2004;432:822–822. doi: 10.1038/432822a. [PubMed] [CrossRef] [Google Scholar]

11. Roe D, Karandikar B, Bonn-Savage N, Gibbins B, Roullet JB. Antimicrobial surface functionalization of plastic catheters by silver nanoparticles. J Antimicrobial Chemother. 2008;61(4):869–876. doi: 10.1093/jac/dkn034. [PubMed] [CrossRef] [Google Scholar]

12. Kokabo M, Sirousazar M, Hassan ZH. PVA–clay nanocomposite hydrogels for wound dressing. Eur Polym J. 2007;43:773–781. doi: 10.1016/j. eurpolymj.2006.11.030. [CrossRef] [Google Scholar]

13. Skalak R, Fox C (1988). Tissue engineering. Proceedings of a workshop held at Granlibakken, Lake Tahoe, California; Liss, New York

ABOUT THE AUTHOR

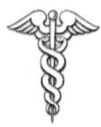

The author qualified as a doctor, MBBS, MS (Master in Surgery), in March 1979 from the prestigious Rohtak Medical College, Rohtak, Haryana (Now known as Pt. B.D. Sharma PGI, Rohtak). He worked as a Senior Resident in the surgery department and then joined the Army Medical Services where he worked as a Graded Surgical Specialist for five years.

He underwent short term training in urology at St Peter's Hospital, London, and one year of urology training at the TMA Pai Rotary Hospital, Mangalore. He trained himself in Laparoscopy at Johnson and Johnson Institute, Mumbai. He underwent training in upper and lower GI Endoscopy from the Asian Institute of Gastroenterology, Hyderabad, and then established a practice in laparoscopic and urology for twenty years.

Later, he joined medical college and served in various positions and is currently functioning as the Professor and Head of Surgery at ESIC Medical College and Hospital, Faridabad, Haryana, India.

He has published more than 85 publications in national and international journals. He has attended many conferences and chaired sessions in most of them. He has organized many regional and state level conferences. He is on the editorial boards of many reputed national and international journals. He has contributed editorials to many of these. He is a lifetime member of many associations and societies like IMA, ASI, FAIGES, USI, Hernia Society of India, ELSA (Singapore) etc.

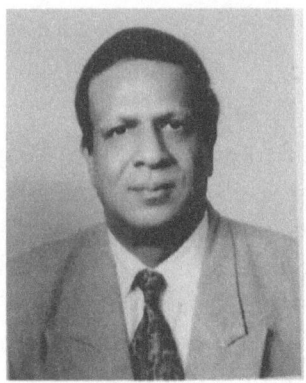